VINTA

# REAL FOODS
## ON A BUDGET

JESSIE HAWKINS

REAL FOODS ON A BUDGET
PUBLISHED BY THISTLE PUBLICATIONS
Franklin, Tennessee
*a division of Vintage Remedies*
www.VintageRemedies.com

ISBN 13: 978-1-938206-00-9

Copyright © 2012 by Jessie Hawkins

All rights reserved. No part of this book may be reproduced or transmitted in any form or by any means, electronic or mechanical, including photocopying and recording, or by any information storage or retrieval system, without permission in writing from the publisher. For requests or permission, please contact Vintage Remedies

*Warning / Disclaimer: This book is intended as a reference volume only, not a medical manual. Every effort has been made to ensure that the information contained herein is complete and accurate. However, you should consult a physician, preferably a physician with experience in natural medicine before altering your diet significantly, particularly if you have preexisting health concerns. Jessie Hawkins and Thistle Publications / Vintage Remedies shall have neither liability nor responsibility to any person or entity regarding any alleged loss, damage or injury as a result of the information presented in this work. If you suspect that you have a medical problem, please do not delay seeking competent help.*

VINTAGE REMEDIES is a registered trademark. All rights reserved.

Library of Congress Cataloging-in-Publication Data

Hawkins, Jessie
    Real Foods on a Budget  / by Jessie Hawkins
    -- 1st Edition


Printed in the United States of America
2012

To my husband Matthew; I am so blessed to have your continued support in my endeavors - for richer or poorer, in sickness and health, in good times and bad. I love you.

# Contents

1. Committed to the Cause 7
2. Eating Like a Peasant 11
3. Go With the Flow 21
4. More Bang for Your Bucks 25
5. New Grocery Lists 31
6. Conventional Stores 35
7. New Grocery Stores 43
8. A Little Help From My Friends 49
9. Stocking Up 53
10. Farm to Table 63
11. Doing it Myself 67
12. Save it for Later 81
13. Allergies and Sensitivities 87
14. Avoiding Burnout 93
15. Quick and Easy Standbys 99

## Tip Number One
## Committed to the Cause

Hippocrates once said, "Let your food be your medicine and your medicine be your food." With today's availability in the grocery store, the only thing modern food is doing to our health is causing health problems. There's definitely nothing positive about consuming refined and processed foods, even when we can obtain them for practically nothing through sales and coupons.

Yet the instant savings can be appealing, especially during times when finances are tight for many families. Who doesn't like getting groceries for half of what they used to pay with sales and coupons? And the savings go much further when we're being more cost effective with entertainment and other areas of life.

However, unlike discounted vacations or movie tickets, cutting corners with our food doesn't result in savings that are long lasting. The final price we pay for these cheap foods ends up being much higher than what we'd pay for healthy, local foods. Why is this?

Our bodies have daily requirements for micronutrients, macronutrients and phytochemicals such as antioxidants. When these needs are not met, our bodies suffer. The results of unhealthy diets include chronic health concerns that are paid for through additional visits to the care provider, days missed from work, lost productivity at the home, and expensive medications or prescriptions. When we add those to the grocery bill, the savings are overshadowed by the additional medical costs these cheap foods dictate.

How many health concerns could realistically be caused by skimping at the grocery store? In the year 2000, the most common cause of unnecessary death and disease in America was poor diet and sedentary lifestyle. A study published in the Journal of the American Medical Association reveals that diet is the second most prominent contributor to mortality in the United States. And mortality isn't the only side effect of a poor diet. Morbidity - or illness - is a serious problem frequently caused by diet.

Obesity, heart disease, type 2 diabetes, and various inflammatory related disorders are all examples of how diet can trigger or worsen health. When we factor in the costs of those serious concerns, the few extra dollars we spend for nutrient dense organic or local foods that can help prevent or eliminate such concerns seem like fantastic bargains!

According to the National Institute of Health, Americans spent over $2.5 trillion on health care costs in 2010, accounting for 17.9% of the nations GDP! This number was significantly higher than it had been and continues to grow. Why? One of the main reasons is a sharp rise in chronic health concerns. The Center for Disease Control estimates that over 75% of those health care costs are for chronic illness, many of which are directly linked to diet.

According to the US Department of Labor, the average American family spent $3,753 in 2009 on groceries and $3,126 on health care expenses. When all health care costs are accounted for, the annual health care costs are over $7,400 per person. Of those expenses, roughly 84% are for physicians visits, hospital visits, prescription drugs and other routine costs.

These numbers just aren't sustainable. And they don't even begin to factor in the emotional costs of premature death, chronic illness, and stress caused by the unpredictability of a medical crisis. I've heard the excuse countless times that additional funds for groceries just are not in the budget. Yet, the rise in chronic health concerns such as recurring ear infections in children, migraine headaches, arthritis, type 2 diabetes, heart disease, and so on, are costly and often focus a reassessment of budgetary priorities.

When prevention is implemented through a real foods diet, and these health care concerns are avoided, the emotional costs are avoided, and the budget is better off, even if a larger portion is allocated to groceries.

So what does that have to do with a book on saving money on the grocery budget? You'll still find many great money saving tips through these pages, but the first step to saving on real foods is to make sure that the priorities are in place. Real foods that can help to prevent these serious health concerns are worth the additional expenditure at the grocery store, and there will be times through this book that I recommend buying something that may be more pricey than what you're used to purchasing. That's because these items are more nutrient dense.

When it all comes together, the best way to save money on groceries is to focus on getting those valuable nutrients into the body. If you can spend a bit more on healthier ingredients - but use fewer ingredients - the overall grocery bill is lower. And, by eliminating diet related health problems, the overall budget is lower, all factors considered.

So as you begin your journey to whole, real foods - or if you've been choosing healthier foods for years - it may be a good idea to reconfigure the whole budget at the get-go to ensure that the ideal amount is dedicated to providing the family with the healthiest food possible. These investments into overall health pay off in measurable ways both immediately and over the years.

## Tip Number Two
## Eat Like a Peasant

Fortunately, raising the grocery budget significantly isn't always necessary. As long as a fair percentage of the overall budget is available for health promoting food, the costs required to feed the family shouldn't be exorbitant, and in my experience, they're not.

And this has been the case throughout history, as the healthiest foods were always the foods of the working class or peasants. Unlike today, when food prices are artificially turned upside down, highly refined and processed foods were generally only available to the very wealthy in times past.

We could use examples through various prominent eras, but perhaps none is so near as the Great Depression, a time period from which we are not too far removed. We all have heard first hand stories from family members that experienced this time of extreme financial hardship.

Some of my fondest childhood memories are in the kitchen and garden with my grandmother, who taught me how to garden and cook. She was born and raised on a rural Alabama farm, so when the Depression hit during her young adult years, she was well equipped with survival skills, as were many of the time.

These families didn't survive this time of financial distress by choosing refined or processed foods. They learned how to adapt using the skills and habits that were common before modern days when we rely on bog box grocery stores and often lack even the most basic of cooking skills.

Meats were luxuries afforded only during celebrations or holidays. Routine meals didn't involve bacon, steaks, chicken, or other meats. They were laden with vegetables, many of which were grown in the backyard. Chickens were too busy laying eggs to be used for a single meal, and canning or otherwise preserving vegetables was a skill shared by every housekeeper.

Now, that's an extreme example, and there are many documented ill effects of the nutrient deficiencies caused by the many families that couldn't manage to obtain enough food, even with those money saving techniques. And as we study various other time periods, there are always instances of those that are not able to obtain enough food to eat, which can be just as dangerous healthwise as an abundance of bad food.

However, the primary point is that this is the first time in history when the average working class diet is not one of the healthiest diets humans can enjoy. A low grocery budget throughout history has dictated a backyard garden, which would have resulted in fresh and local vegetables and fruits which were all grown organically until just a few decades ago. Later in this book, we'll see why local and organic foods are the most nutrient dense foods available.

A low grocery budget has historically meant that there wasn't enough money to buy refined sugar or meats to enjoy two or three times a day. Low budgets have meant vegetarian protein sources, large intake of low glycemic carbohydrates, and limited healthy fats.

Yet now we have the whole thing upside down, where a low budget means the only thing available at the grocery store is refined and processed high glycemic carbohydrates, fake fats and cheap, mass produced unhealthy animal meats.

So my first tip for getting a real foods diet on a realistic budget is to eat like a peasant. Not a modern day peasant, but a historical working-class family that only bought refined treats for birthdays or holidays and consumed fresh vegetable laden diets on most average days. What does this diet look like in the twenty-first century?

**Realistic Portions**

One feature of a restricted budget in times past is that there was not an abundance of excess food, so overeating wasn't as easy. When we prepare large, unrealistic portions at the table, overeating is a concern. When there isn't excess food to waste, it's not a concern. I'm not merely suggesting that we all eat less. Rather, prepare the correct portions for the best diet and to maximize savings. Modern Americans throw away large amounts of food every day.

This begins at the grocery store. How often do we have to clean out our pantries and refrigerator? When we do that, how much food do we throw away that was never prepared? How much of the budget does that take up? Chances are - a significant portion.

With very few exceptions - which we will cover in later chapters - I only buy what I know my family will eat within the next week or two. I don't buy what I want them to eat or what would be fun to play around with in the kitchen. I don't buy what's on sale. I buy what we will eat; nothing more, nothing less. The grocery store isn't the place for optimism; it's a place for realism.

This eliminates the problem of having to go through the fridge and toss what we didn't consume because when I buy what I wish we ate instead of what I know we'll eat, we never eat it all. This is especially true during the transition to real foods when the family isn't accustomed to the different grocery items just yet. Don't stock up on what you want them to eat, stock up on what you know they'll eat, even if it's not what you want them to eat. As long as you're making steps in the right direction and continue making progress, you'll get there eventually.

I also use a first in, first out system in the fridge to avoid waste. For example, we get our eggs from a CSA we participate in (more on that in a few chapters) and get several dozen once a month. Sometimes we haven't finished the previous month's eggs, but by putting the new eggs in the back, with the old eggs in the front, I've not tossed an egg in years. They're all eaten and never go bad.

Likewise, when preparing a meal, I don't cook more than my family will eat. I prepare foods for them three times a day, so I'm pretty familiar with how much of any food they will eat, and prepare the exact amount of food for 6 realistic portions at each meal. This provides enough for all of us with nothing left over. We don't have leftover nights, and don't have to worry about how to creatively get the family to enjoy leftovers. We don't eat leftovers because we don't make leftovers.

**Stocking Basics**

Another important habit is to keep the basics stocked in the kitchen. Were we preparing these foods from our backyard harvest, long lasting staples would always be available in the pantry. However, with modern purchasing habits, these may not always come from our own kitchens. So keeping these things on hand ensures that we actually use and maximize the groceries we buy. How often have you had all but one ingredient for a favorite recipe but by the time you restock that ingredient, others have gone bad?

There are certain foods I make sure we always have fully stocked. Usually this means I'm buying it in bulk or buying extra to ensure that we don't even get low in these supplies. This enables me to prepare standby meals without having to run to the store for last minute items that usually cost more at the local grocery.

**Ingredient Substitutions**

Simultaneously, learning how to play around with your recipes will also enable you to maximize your budget and reduce waste. Even with a fully stocked pantry, there could always be an ingredient that may be forgotten when prepping for the week's menu. Instead of making a quick trip to the local grocer that may be more expensive than your usual standby, learn how to adjust the recipes to substitute other ingredients.

Many of my favorite cookbooks from the 1800s and early 1900s contain lists of common substitutions to enable busy cooks to quickly grab another option when the recommended ingredient is not available. I've included one at the end of this chapter for your convenience.

**Unconventional Meals**

Another habit used by regular people through history is to eat to get nourishment, not to get the modern standard of the multi-course meal. We have so many societal expectations about mealtime and many of them are in direct contradiction to what's healthiest for our bodies.

Breakfast doesn't always have to include fruit, bacon, eggs and baked goods. It can include beans, vegetables, or crackers if that's what's on hand and provides the necessary nutrients. Dinner time doesn't always have to include a salad, meat, and three vegetables. It can be a salad and sandwich combo or an assortment of veggies. My favorite childhood meal was at my grandmother's house. We'd look forward to the night we had vegetables for dinner, which included black eyed peas, creamed corn, dinner rolls, sliced tomatoes, and maybe some potatoes. She prepared the peas and corn from a harvest purchased from local farmers every summer and prepared them all at once, freezing individual portions. This favorite meal of ours took her just a few minutes to prepare and it wasn't until we were older that we realized this was her daily standby for routine meals. By today's standards, the meal was unconventional, but it was affordable, quick, easy, and, most importantly, healthy - packed with phytonutrients, antioxidants, micronutrients and micronutrients.

When we get out of the modern confines of our daily meal expectations, the options for healthy and affordable meals are limitless! Try playing around with various options and foods at different times of the day to find out what works best for your family's needs and your schedule.

**Become a Foodie**

Professional chefs and foodies alike can agree on the one thing that makes a gourmet meal special, the quality of the ingredients. Some of the best meals are composed of a few simple but spectacular ingredients . By focusing on quality - fresh local tomatoes and organic fresh basil, for example - amazing meals can be tossed together with fewer ingredients. This provides more room in the budget for higher quality ingredients and because the meal doesn't rely on additives for flavor, the robust flavor of fresh, local food elevates the quality and nutrition in your routine meals.

This can be combined with other techniques in this chapter. By rethinking the types of meals you serve, you may be able to reduce the ingredient list for a dinnertime meal from about 20 to 3-4. As long as you're focusing on a variety of foods throughout the year and these foods are healthy, nutrient dense real foods, the overall nutritional quality of your meals will be dramatically increased, and the overall culinary quality will get a boost as well.

## Vegetable Proteins / Meatless Meals

With conventional foods, butter substitutes, meats and other animal products are affordable, so changing to a real foods diet can seem to be expensive at first, unless those habits are changed. Traditional diets were not so heavily dependent upon animal products, which were used less frequently in the average home.

Instead, for protein, vegetable products were prominent parts of the diet. Beans, which are easy to grow in the backyard, can be purchased in bulk, and are easily stored for long periods of time with little to no special storage requirements, make an ideal addition to the real foods diet. In addition to providing lots of heart healthy vegetable based protein, beans and legumes are extremely affordable.

Depending on your current diet, reducing animal products might mean cutting back to twice a day or it may mean having meatless days each week. One easy way to begin is to implement a "Meatless Monday," which simply means focusing on vegetable based meals once a week. Once that is mastered, additional days can be added, as desired.

Cutting back on fats like oils and butters can also help reduce the "rich" foods in the diet, eliminating a large expense from the grocery bill.

## Pantry / Fridge Challenge

One of the best ways to get started is to undertake a pantry/fridge challenge. This will help you clean out your fridge and pantry without tossing the majority of what you have. Then, it will be freshly cleared for your new start with real foods on a budget.

It's simple to undertake this challenge. An extreme version includes only using the foods you already have on hand for up to a month without buying anything else. If you have a packed pantry and fridge, that may be an option, but otherwise, it's probably best to modify the challenge for an average family.

The way I do the pantry/fridge challenge is to begin by emptying the whole pantry out onto the kitchen table. Then I begin making a list of the meals I can make with those ingredients. If I need any additional ingredients, I buy only the things I will need to finish off everything I have in the pantry first - with the exception of the items I buy in bulk. For a few weeks, the grocery bill is very small while we enjoy the foods we've already purchased instead of trashing them later when they expire. Then I start afresh with a clean pantry and clean fridge.

## Substitution List

Baking powder (1 teaspoon) = 1/4 teaspoon baking soda plus 5/8 teaspoon cream of tartar

Brown sugar (1 cup) = 1 cup organic sugar + 2 t molasses

Buttermilk (1 cup) = 1 cup yogurt

Cream of Tarter (1 teaspoon) = 1 T lemon juice

Egg = 1 banana or 1 T agar flakes mixed into 1 T water

Gelatin = agar agar flakes (equal parts)

Herbs, fresh (1 tablespoon) = 1 t dried herbs

Meat = beans (equal parts)

Oil, for baking = equal parts applesauce

Oil, for cooking = veggie stock, vinegar

Sour Cream (1 cup) = 7/8 cup sour milk plus 3 T butter

Wine, red (1 cup) = 13 T water + 3 T lemon juice + 1 t sugar OR pomegranate juice OR 1 cup water plus 1 t balsamic vinegar

Wine, white = equal parts veggie stock or apple juice

## Tip Number Three
## Go With the Flow

One of the best pieces of advice I can give for healthy eating within a reasonable budget is to eat with the seasons. Seasonal eating is becoming a trendy notion due to the local eating movement, but it has budgetary benefits in addition to the health benefits.

Prior to the widespread availability of stored food that entered the scene in the early 1900s, seasonal eating was the norm for thousands of generations. And it's a very healthy and nutritious way to eat.

When we consume foods when they are ripe, we're getting the most nutrient dense foods. As food is harvested, the nutrient content stops developing. The longer it takes to get our food from the farm to our table, the greater the loss of nutrients. So when we purchase foods closer to their harvest date, we can ensure the most nutrient dense food available.

Additionally, eating with the seasons can benefit our bodies. In the summer, when it's hot outside and we are concerned about hydration, the foods that are ripe are some of the most hydrating fruits and vegetables we consume. Things like tomatoes and watermelon provide the additional hydration we need during these hotter months. They are also generally consumed as-is. This eliminates the need to spend warm summer days in the kitchen standing over a hot stove, which is further heating our already warm homes. Instead, the foods are ready to eat with little preparation and little added heat. These summer foods are also generally either consumed quickly after harvest or preserved through canning or dehydrating for use later in the year.

As the fall approaches, the foods that are ripe have longer shelf lives, without additional storage requirements. Things like potatoes and apples can stay fresh for months - long enough to get us through the cold winter until the next harvest. Additionally, many of these fall foods are cooked - often combined with meats for warming stews and soups. These help to warm our bodies and are foods that tend to increase body fat content slightly - something that would have been beneficial prior to modern heating devices.

Throughout the winter, these stored foods are enjoyed, and in some locations lettuces, carrots, onions and similar root vegetables can still be harvested throughout some of the colder months. This combines perfectly with the stews and soups prepared with those stored vegetables to keep our bodies nourished and provide some additional micronutrients.

As warmer months approach, the spring harvest is packed with liver supportive detoxification foods such as asparagus and additional greens. These foods are perfect for helping to lose that winter weight and prepare the body for the hotter summer-y months. They also support the liver, enabling the body to detoxify any toxins absorbed from staying cooped up indoors for several months.

Then, when the hotter months arrive, the cycle begins again with the hydrating fruits and vegetables. This pattern was perfectly designed to support our bodies through the seasons, providing us with the exact nutrients we need when we need them.

While we don't necessarily deal with some of those issues anymore due to modern conveniences, the benefits of seasonal eating go beyond the seasonal changes our bodies experience.

Consuming the foods that are fresh and in season means that the length of time between the farm to your table is reduced. This means the foods will be more nutrient dense, making each meal healthier. It also eliminates the waste produced from transportation as most of our modern foods travel thousands of miles to get to our tables. It's been estimated that we indirectly consume much more gas to get these foods to our table then we directly put into our cars each year.

In addition to the health benefits, seasonal eating has great savings potential. When these foods are available from the local suppliers, the supply is huge, thus the price is more reasonable. At the farmer's markets, you can usually get large supplies of fresh produce for much cheaper when there's an abundance of that product. And when local suppliers are packed with supply, grocers that buy locally will also have deep discounts during that time of year.

If you've ever tried to find some good organic strawberries in January, you know how difficult that can be. However, in July, there's no problem finding organic strawberries - often in bulk - for a fraction of the price. Enjoy food when its in season and stock up on your favorites while they're discounted!

## Tip Number Four
## More Bang for Your Bucks

So the next important key reminder in healthier eating on a reasonable budget is to pack the most nutrients into each piece of food. Buying cheap food isn't really saving money when you realize how little there is in that food to sustain your health.

Our bodies require certain levels of nutrients each day. We need a minimum intake of a wide variety of micronutrients, macronutrients, and phytochemicals. Micronutrients are the tiny nutrients in foods - the vitamins and minerals. Macronutrients are the larger nutrients - fats, carbohydrates and proteins. Phytochemicals include the antioxidants, prebiotics, and other substances in food that are not specifically classified as micro- or macronutrients, but our bodies require them for optimal health. Many phytochemicals have yet to even be discovered and identified.

These necessary components are not available in laboratory produced foods. Food dyes, additives, hydrogenated fats and processed sugars don't provide vitamins and minerals. They can be ingested into the body - and the body can even hold on to them, allowing them to hinder optimal development and health. But they don't provide those necessary tools we need to stay healthy.

So if we look at our bodies like we look at our cars. Let's say we have a required level of necessary substances - fuel, washing fluid, coolant, oil. Our bodies have required levels of iron, magnesium, B complex vitamins, healthy fats, carbohydrates. When these levels are not maintained, something will go wrong. The car may not start, it may overheat, or it may suffer severe damage. Our bodies may become sluggish, they may develop a wide variety of chronic complaints, or we may suffer severe damage. These levels have to be maintained through regular intake of nutrient dense foods.

Processed foods that don't provide those requirements are literally wasting our money. They're causing harm to our bodies, without providing any of the necessary tools to reverse that harm and achieve optimal health.

Consuming a bag of colorful sugary candies will not provide any of those nutrients. Neither will a bowl full of colorful O shaped flavored cereal. But they will both contribute to diabetes, obesity, heart disease and other complaints that will increase the body's requirements of protective nutrients such as antioxidants and various minerals. So, to be more specific, intake of these processed foods not only wastes money, it costs more money - money that is spent in supplements to build back up the body's stores of necessary nutrients, money that is spent in prescription drugs to treat the health concerns, and money that is spent on doctor's visits to diagnose and monitor those health concerns. And that does not even mention the money lost to missed days at work and decreased productivity at home, or the missed enjoyment from family time due to decreased health.

Real foods, however are packed with nutrients that maintain optimal bodily health. So, purchasing a selection of fruit for morning smoothies may take a minute or two longer than tossing together a bowl of cereal, but that time is an investment into the future, as the benefits of increased energy levels and optimal health pay off. Additionally, it may cost a dollar or two more at the grocery store, but we're saving annually through decreased medical costs and increased productivity.

So, to stretch your budget, getting the most out of each food purchase is essential. Choosing foods that will replenish the levels of nutrients our bodies require will pack the most into each purchase, stretching your dollar further. Avoiding all processed foods and ingredients is the best way to make that happen.

**Even More Bang for Your Buck**

Additionally, when comparing conventional foods to local and/or organic foods, you can pack even more nutrients into each meal by choosing organic. When compared directly, organic foods contain far more micronutrients and antioxidants than the conventional option, enabling you to get the most for each piece of produce you purchase.

For example, a recent study compared four nutrients and a toxin in conventional and organic produce. The organic produce had 27% more vitamin C, 21% more iron, 29% more magnesium, 14% more phosphorus and 15% fewer nitrates.

**Meal Planning**

Another important way to save on groceries is to focus on the specific meals you're going to prepare and only buy those ingredients. Sure, meal planning is something that is touted everywhere for a variety of reasons, but the primary reason I recommend the practice is because it can eliminate the habit of purchasing foods and ingredients that we don't end up using.

The best way to waste money at the grocery store is to purchase foods we don't consume. It wouldn't matter if those foods were nutrient dense or not - they go from the store to our food storage locations to the trash or composter. They take up valuable space in our grocery budgets, valuable space in our pantries or refrigerators and then increase our trash output.

When we plan our meals, I can customize the grocery list for those meals. Only the ingredients we need and plan on consuming are purchased and nothing additional makes it onto the list, taking up valuable space.

Another option for this step is to become more creative in the kitchen, substituting ingredients in favorite recipes for what is on hand. When using the seasonal eating method, it may be more cost effective to skip the meal planning and only purchase what's in season at the farmer's market. However, if we stick to recipes with very specific ingredient lists, we end up spending more at the grocery stores buying the exact foods that fit into that recipe. Instead, play around with the ingredients on sale and substitute those in your family's favorite recipes. They key here is that you should make good use of your culinary skills and be prepared to enjoy the experiments that don't prove to be as successful as others.

**Maximizing Portions**

Finally, combining the various foods for the meal can alter the cost of a meal significantly. Again, looking at each meal as an opportunity to provide the variety of nutrients needed in a day. Serving a protein dense meal that is low in micronutrients won't be the best way to accomplish that - especially since protein rich foods are often more costly than micronutrient dense foods.

For example, a traditional breakfast with bacon, eggs and toast with butter or jam could be improved financially and nutritionally by reducing the amount of bacon and adding some fresh fruits or homemade granola bars.

A dinner that features a steak with a side of asparagus could be healthier and less costly if the steak was smaller and the meal also contained another vegetable side or two.

By selecting ingredients that are nutrient dense, arranging them in meals so they complement each other, ensuring a wide variety of nutrients throughout the day without the need for excess food, and purchasing only the foods we're going to eat, the weekly grocery budget is much more manageable and flexible - without the need to clip coupons and monitor sales to buy foods that won't nourish our bodies and foods we may not even want to consume.

## Tip Number Five
## New Grocery Lists

Many healthy changes in the diet and budget begin with a change in overall habits. For example, if you've spent years consuming a traditional processed diet, you've probably also spent many years buying the same items from the grocery store trip after trip.

Most grocery store items are not ingredients but prepared foods ready to simply be heated or stirred before serving. Meals in a box fill the aisles, and some items come fully prepared so that all we do is open a box or twist the lid off a jar and call it a meal.

When those same grocery lists are converted to organic and healthier options, the grocery bill skyrockets. Processed toaster pastries may be cheap, especially with a coupon, but organic hydrogenated oil-free toaster pastries with real fruit are easily more expensive than driving through for breakfast!

This difference in price perpetuates the myth that healthy food is always more expensive than conventional food. Real foods shouldn't be that much more expensive than conventional food, and with a healthy grocery budget, there shouldn't be any significant annual change in overall expenditures for a real foods diet.

The key is to change the grocery list and eliminate the processed foods such as boxed cereal, packaged goods and prepared foods - whether they are organic or not. Processed foods are still processed foods, even if the ingredients are grown without pesticides. They're not going to be healthy for us, even if they are void of the additives and carcinogens found in conventional processed foods.

However, mastering this habit can be frustrating, especially at first. Once you begin consciously avoiding the processed and packaged foods at the grocery store, you find that your favorite grocery store actually has very little food!

Instead of spending extra on these foods, choose basic ingredients for your favorite foods. This enables you to make a healthier food with real foods, minus the additives. It will also result in substantial savings on the grocery bill.

The best way to begin is to take your usual grocery list and go through each item individually. Look at the major ingredients in each item and write those on your list instead.

For example, if you've been buying organic cookie dough, change the list to flour, sugar, eggs, chocolate chips, vanilla extract. At the first trip, you may end up spending a touch more if you don't already stock these basics in your home. But you probably already have most, if not all, of those ingredients in your house. And per cookie, the savings are significant.

To save time, make large batches of cookie dough at once. With a few minutes one day, you can have a supply of frozen cookie dough ready to go when you need it next, and enjoy your savings on both time and money over the next few months.

Another important change in your overall grocery list is to eliminate the items that are not beneficial. One great example is the many drink items we purchase. Fruit juices, flavored drinks, sodas, flavored milks - the list of these drinks can go on and on, but there is no health benefit to any of these items. Sure, you can get an additive and pesticide free option, but there still won't be any significant health benefit worth obtaining through this purchase. However, when you omit these items from the list, replacing them with fresh water, teas, and whole fruit and veggie smoothies, the grocery total is reduced and overall health is improved.

There are many similar items in the list that just don't need to be replaced with ingredients and can be omitted altogether. As you evaluate the list, keep an eye out for the items that can be removed instead of perfected.

## Tip Number Six
## Conventional Stores

The best deals on real foods are not usually found at conventional stores, but I'd be kidding if I pretended that we never stop by a store for a quick grocery run. And sometimes, a conventional store - especially in winter - may be the only reasonable option.

So when you find yourself at a regular grocery store, keep a few things in mind. First, if you have health food store options, don't shy away from those. If you're already buying real foods, it's a myth that the natural store chains are more expensive. Sure, if you load up on the gourmet cheeses and steaks, you'll spend a fortune, but for the regular staples, you might be surprised!

Most of the routine purchases we make at a big grocery store are available in a generic option at the health food store, which is available for a fraction of the name brand cost at a conventional grocery store. This is especially the case with dried foods such as lentils, beans, and rice. It's also true for nut butters, jams and similar items. So, when there's an option, I generally opt for the natural food store to get the best deals on these basics.

However, at conventional stores, there are still savings to be found. If you don't have a natural food store nearby or the local produce options are limited, there are ways to get the most important organics without going broke.

One method is to always check out the dirty dozen list put out annually by the Environmental Working Group. This list can be found on their website at www.EWG.com and I've included the 2011 results at the end of this chapter. The dirty dozen is a list of 12 foods that are most likely to contain the highest levels of pesticides, based on testing they conduct annually. If conventional versions of these 12 foods are replaced with organic versions, a significant reduction in pesticide consumption will be the result.

However, keep in mind that the list only covers pesticides. Sometimes there are foods that are considered to be acceptable in the conventional variety that I wouldn't purchase without an organic label. Nonetheless, if a family only consumed 12 organic produce items and consumed conventional varieties of everything else, these would be the 12 to buy for the most benefit.

When the cost for organic produce is so much higher, splurging on those 12 items will get the most value for the money, and it's not as big of an ordeal to save on the conventional produce. Before you decide not to get organic varieties of all major produce items, however, don't forget the More Bang for Your Bucks chapter!

Here's an overview of what I usually buy at regular grocery stores. I've included all of the major stores I stop at on a regular basis. Not all of them are close to me, but I make the drive to stock up on these essentials regularly.

During the summer, I find that I usually don't buy anything but dried goods and paper goods at grocery stores, but during the winter or when preparing for a big party or holiday, I find myself there more often.

What you find to be worthwhile at these stores will vary, but I've included what I consider to be the best deals on real foods at each popular chain. If you don't have one of these near you, you'll know what to stock up on when you do come across one. And if you do have these options, you'll want to keep an eye out for these bargains!

**What I buy:**

There are some staples that I just can't get from my CSAs, co-ops and farmers' market. So I usually stock up on these through grocery stores. When the savings are substantial, I've listed those items below:

**Trader Joe's Market**

**Arborio Rice** - Most bulk options don't carry this rice, which is great for risotto - my favorite gluten free comfort food.

**Candy** - Yes, we do buy candy sometimes, and when we do, we like to stick with natural sugars, colors and flavors. Here I can find a variety of safe candy for a fraction of what I pay elsewhere - it's priced much like regular candy at a regular grocery store. So if it's Christmas, Easter or a birthday and you want to splurge on something, here's where to find decent treats at a decent price.

**Cheeses** - They have a surprisingly large cheese selection, including some basics like shredded cheddar and some fun finds like raw milk flavored cheeses. The prices are always great and the milk is always hormone free. If you regularly use shredded cheeses in your meals or if you like serving a fun cheese plate at times, here's a great place for variety and savings.

**Chips** - We use tortilla chips for a variety of things and I can find chips using organic corn here for about the same price I would pay for conventional chips elsewhere.

**Handmade Tortillas** - I like to make my own tortillas so they're healthier, but I stock up on these amazing handmade tortillas and keep them in the freezer for quick and easy burrito nights.

**Paper Goods** - My tissues, toilet paper, and paper towels all come from Trader Joes. It's the only place I can find high quality recycled paper goods for what I'd pay for conventional goods at another store. It's not that scratchy, useless paper towel or toilet paper roll that you find elsewhere, which only contains a small percentage of recycled materials. These are great and very eco-friendly.

**Pet Food** - I don't make my pet's food, but I do feel she should have something more natural than just whatever's available. So I get it here. Like the other items on this list, I can get something healthier for about what I pay for regular stuff elsewhere.

**Snacks** - Dried fruits, nuts, fruit leathers and other healthy snacks are much more reasonably priced here. I don't make any of these items at home and don't necessarily want to buy them in bulk. My family does enjoy them, however, so we usually get them here - there's a large variety of trail mix materials and usually plenty of organic options.

**Sodas** - Like the candy, this is a treat for a birthday or holiday, but when we splurge, this is where we do it. The store brand is packaged in glass bottles and priced much less than what we can find elsewhere for natural sodas.

**Costco**

**Organic Spinach** - In the produce section, I can usually find a huge container of pre-washed spinach for about the same price 2 regular bunches would cost me at any other store, which makes breakfast smoothies a snap and I save a few bucks on my weekly spinach bill!

**Healthier Pre-packaged Lunchbox Treats** - During our busy travel season, I like to prepare the kids' lunches before I leave town. These are not snacks I'd usually buy, but if I'm going to spend on a pre-packaged item, this is the place to do it. I can get organic fruit gummies, crackers, healthier chips and granola bars by my favorite brands for less. And with four kids, the larger sized boxes still go pretty quickly.

**Olive Oil** - Every spring, Costco has a supply of high quality, fresh olive oil that was produced from the previous late fall harvest in Europe. It's some of the freshest and best olive oil I've purchased and the price is very reasonable. I usually stock up on 10-12 bottles of this oil to last the year.

**Whole Foods**

**Local Produce (in season)** - Whole Foods usually buys produce from local farmers whenever possible. So during the spring and summer months, this means I can find produce from my favorite farmers throughout the week, not just at the Saturday market. And the prices are usually close to what I'd pay at the market - sometimes lower.

**Dry Goods** - What I don't buy in bulk, I get from Whole Foods. They have a wide variety of dried goods such as rice, beans and grains, and the store brand is priced very reasonably for organic staples.

**Regular Chain Grocery Stores**

I don't usually find any great deals on healthy food at regular grocery stores unless they are discontinuing items and they're significantly discounted. Even in those cases, it's usually a semi-processed item made from organic ingredients. When I end up at a regular grocery store, I know I'm going to spend more on my meal, but it saves time being the closest store to my home.

**What I don't usually buy at a grocery store:**

**Fresh Produce** - With my regular CSAs, I can get local and organic produce for less. If I'm going to buy something, I usually try to stick with Whole Foods for local farms or Costco if I can get organic at a savings.

**Meats** - Again, I usually get this from a CSA to avoid the risks of large-scale produced meat products. Exceptions: When I run out of local eggs, I can find a local farmer at Whole Foods and sometimes my husband likes to grab something to grill at the last minute, so we get a steak or two at Whole Foods - again for the local factor. When we do cheat on these rules, we always end up spending more, usually much more.

The 2011 Dirty Dozen by the Environmental Working Group:

1. Apples
2. Celery
3. Strawberries
4. Peaches
5. Spinach
6. Nectarines - imported
7. Grapes - imported
8. Sweet bell peppers
9. Potatoes
10. Blueberries - domestic
11. Lettuce
12. Kale / collard greens

## Tip Number Seven
## New Grocery Stores

So, if I'm not getting my food from a regular grocery store, where do I get it? My shopping habits are often scheduled by appointments with farmers and by the natural seasons of the year. By doing this, I always get the most for each dollar and the bonus is that I'm getting the healthiest foods around. My "grocery stores" include:

**Farmers**

I buy most of my foods directly from farmers. By getting to know my local farmers, we develop relationships that enable me to see my food produced from start to finish. The farmers that raise our meats welcome us out year round so we can see the hatchlings beginning to grow, the cows wondering through the fields or the chickens laying eggs. We know they use solar energy fences to protect the chickens and that the coops have wheels on the bottom so the chickens can move about throughout their large outdoors space finding bugs in a safe area.

We visit our produce farmers and watch them planting new crops, knowing we can begin the countdown for the bounty of some of our favorites. We watch them maintaining the crops and know how they care for them naturally and organically. With this relationship, we're able to know exactly where our food comes from and that it meets our standards of quality - which transition to standards of health. And because we're buying direct, we get to eliminate the various "middle man" sources in between us and our food - such as the grocery store.

## CSAs

One of the best ways to purchase directly from a farmer is through a Community Supported Agriculture agreement. CSA for short, this agreement is a benefit to both the consumer and the farmer. By agreeing to purchase a share from the farmer through a predetermined season, the farmer knows he/she has buyers for their products and the consumer knows he/she has a fantastic source of locally grown, healthy food each week or month of the harvest season.

In the early days, CSAs were seen by some to be a bit of a risk. The agreement includes a fixed price for the year, but the content of the box or basket varies by the harvest season and weather. Sometimes the box would be packed with goodies, while other weeks had much smaller harvests. However, most CSA farmers now plan ahead to ensure that those boxes will be consistently filled each week or month with fresh produce. The content will still vary - sometimes I get lots of strawberries from my farmers each week, but in other years, I only get a few small containers due to weather conditions. However, I always get a box filled with something fresh - usually produce that has been harvested hours before.

There are many different CSAs available. The standard is a summer CSA that goes through late spring until early fall. Typically 26 weeks in our area, this CSA option is ideal for all families. We begin with strawberries and asparagus and finish with pumpkin and winter squashes. In between we enjoy dozens of amazing foods from the traditional tomatoes and corn to heirloom varieties of nontraditional favorites. You can usually also choose the size of your share. If you have a larger family, try a full share, which is usually a half bushel of produce each week. You could also try a quarter bushel of produce a week or a half bushel every other week - depending on the arrangement the farmers have set up.

Many farmers now also offer winter CSAs, which enable you to continue enjoying the harvest through the winter with winter hardy crops such as lettuces, carrots and radishes - usually grown in a greenhouse. These are ideal for those winter celebrations such as Thanksgiving and Christmas when we want to enjoy an abundance of healthy foods, but the harvest season has past.

Other CSAs include meat CSAs, which provide a regular share of various kinds of prepared meats from chicken to eggs, steaks and pork. Our farmer allows us to customize the share so that we only get the meats our family will enjoy through the month. The kids love visiting the farm where the animals are raised and I'm happy to see how well cared for they are.

Herb CSAs are also newer versions of CSAs cropping up. With these, the farmer is usually an herbalist and grows a wide variety of plants, then makes various herbal preparations from the harvest. By signing up, you can get a supply of fresh or dried herbs plus several balms, salves or extracts from the herbalist based on the current harvest. It's a great way to save money on your natural remedies if you're comfortable with the preparations and plants used, as well as the knowledge and experience of the herbalist.

**Farmers' Markets**

Farmers' markets are my absolute favorite grocery stores. Sure, they're not open 24/7 and I usually have to take time out of my Saturday morning to grocery shop, but the experience is well worth it, and so are the savings.

At our local market, I can stroll through the various stalls and get milk, vegetables, fruit, baked goods featuring local ingredients, meats, honey, and many other random items that feature local or upcycled materials and ingredients. I can find birthday gifts, all of my kitchen perishables, and various additional treats as well.

However, the best part is that I get to directly interact with the farmers and artisans. Instead of getting my items from a big box store where I never know exactly where it came from, I can chat with our farmers about assorted recent events, learn how their summer harvest is coming along, and discover other interesting and unique tidbits about my food. That alone makes the experience worthwhile.

But in addition to that, eliminating the middle-men means that they can offer me the best prices for my food because they're selling it direct. It usually also means they can sell their food or products for more than what the large scale grocery stores pay, so we both win.

Additionally, I'm getting food that's about as fresh and local as it can be aside from growing it in my backyard. Usually my produce was harvested the same day or the day before, and the short distance from the farm to my table means that it's nutrient dense food, just like I'd grow it if I had the time.

Not all vendors at a farmers' market will provide organic, semi-organic or local foods. At our larger market, I'll often find bananas in March, and I live in Tennessee where bananas are never in season! So, you'll want to take advantage of the opportunity to meet the farmers, learn about their habits, and make sure they provide the kind of food you want to feed your family. It takes a little extra time at first, but once you develop those relationships, it's like a little reunion when you come back to grocery shop each week!

**Pick Your Own Farms**

The next best thing to growing your food is to visit a pick your own farm. Many farmers allow families to come into their farms and harvest their own crops. This is a fantastic activity for the kids and is a great way to get some savings. By participating in the workload, the price for the harvest you pick yourself is usually a fraction of what it would cost to get it directly, even at the market.

We love our annual trips to various local farms for household staples. One of my kids' favorite is a local blueberry patch. We've gone to the same patch every summer since the oldest was a toddler. We get up early to avoid the hottest part of the day, and spend hours picking blueberries to fill our buckets. Then we break for lunch and read a book about blueberries while enjoying a picnic in the grass. With 4-5 full buckets, I rarely spend much, but we have enough for the year. We head home. The kids are exhausted and enjoy reading or napping while I wash the berries. For the next few days we have blueberry buckle, blueberry pancakes, blueberry smoothies, and just about everything blueberry you can imagine. Then I freeze the rest individually on cookie sheets. Once frozen, I package in freezer bags with the air removed. For the rest of the year, we have organic, local berries available for smoothies, pancakes, and whatever else we want to make.

Berries are one of the most common products at pick your own farms, but you can also often find peaches, corn, tomatoes, and other summery snacks. Just ask around at the farmers' market and you'll be surprised at what's available!

## Tip Number Eight
## A Little Help From My Friends

In addition to expanding outside of the local grocery options, with a little help, you can also obtain huge savings on dry goods by combining your buying power with that of a few friends. Whole foods co-ops provide a great way to save significantly on groceries and have been used by health conscious families for decades.

With a real foods co-op, you don't shop weekly or monthly as you would through a regular grocery store or even a CSA. Instead, you combine a list of what you'll need for 3-12 months at a time and buy in bulk. When you combine that list with lists from like minded families, you've got a sizable order!

With this increased buying power, you're able to obtain significant discounts - usually around 50% off - from wholesale suppliers. While the initial investment is high, and the planning can be time consuming, the end result is year round savings on the staples you know your family will use.

I use co-ops to obtain all of my dry goods such as wheat, barley, rice, oats, and so on. I also use them for any personal products I don't make myself. During our busy traveling season - which runs from mid spring to mid fall or nearly half of the year - I don't always have the time to make products at the quality I prefer for my family. So, I can still enjoy the safety and security of natural products at a savings by planning ahead and buying in bulk.

Most co-ops require some volunteer work in exchange for the discounted goods. When you go in with a group, someone has to maintain the order, place the order, invest in the order, receive the order and divide the order. With a small group of 5-10 families, this can consume a day or two easily. With a large group of a few dozen families, this can be a part time job! If all families volunteer some time managing the overhead work, the work and savings can be enjoyed by all. When families don't volunteer their time to assist with the associated work, many co-ops charge a handling fee to cover the time investment.

Some of my favorite co-ops include:

Azure Standard - They provide grains and other dry goods to most states on the western side of the US.

Frontier co-op - Frontier provides name brand essential oils, herbs, personal care products, dry goods and other items to the whole country.

Something Better Natural Foods - They provide dry goods to the midwest and east coast.

To begin a co-op in your area, you can contact one of the companies above and set up an account or you can ask about a contact person in your area that has an existing account. You may also find groups that order from several different coops in your area, providing you a larger array of items by contacting local homeschool or childbirth focused groups for like minded families.

## Tip Number Nine
## Stocking Up

Generally speaking, I don't recommend buying more than you plan on consuming within the next week or two when trying to stay on a budget. However, due to the dramatic savings of fresh produce in season, especially when combined with the health benefits of local and organic food, sometimes it's best to stock up.

For example, during mid July to mid August, tomatoes are usually reduced significantly at the local farmers' market due to overabundance of the harvest. Most farmers are happy to sell boxes packed with the uglier tomatoes that are not as presentable for regular sales but still taste fine. These are perfect for use in homemade tomato sauce, which can be thrown together during a lazy summer afternoon.

Likewise, when we go to pick your own farms, we usually stock up on that item for the year, enjoying fresh produce for a week or two, then freezing or otherwise storing the rest in the method that we use most often - usually freezing - for that particular food.

In these situations, buying more than you plan to use in a week or two is a benefit because you save so much by stocking up during these times. As long as you prepare them for storage correctly, there won't be a problem with using all of your excess before the expiration time, which results in benefits throughout the year.

Additionally, there are routine dry goods that can be purchased in bulk for increased savings. Through various co-ops, you can usually obtain wheat, rice, oats, and other dry grains in 25-50 pounds bags for about the cost of 10 pounds packaged in smaller containers at the grocery store.

Upfront costs also include a large plastic bin to store the grains; this protects them from bugs, moisture, and other potential contamination hazards that could cost you the whole purchase. But these bins are also inexpensive and can be reused multiple times over the years.

I usually buy my grains in bulk about once a year in the same order. I rarely spend more than a month's grocery budget, so the investment isn't too huge, and we never have to worry about not having flours or grains for meals. That being said, many flours can go rancid, so if you're buying a year's worth at a time, you'll want to keep your flours in the fridge or even in the freezer to prolong freshness.

Nuts and oils can also be purchased in bulk but I don't recommend buying more than about 4-6 months worth at a time, and even that amount should always be stored in the fridge, which usually means an additional fridge for storing food is a must. You'll have to do the math to determine whether or not it's worth it to invest in a second fridge and keep it running through the months to save a little on nuts and oils. If not stored in the fridge, it's wise to stick with no more than 2-3 months of nuts and oils at a time. They go rancid quickly, and the whole batch can be ruined when that occurs.

Many bulk coops will also provide various mixes and packaged foods at a discount. Usually those are not worth the savings, especially when they're items you can make at home in minutes - like granola bars or cookie mixes. So the best dry goods for coops are the grains, flavorings such as extracts and salts, and beans, which last years in regular storage.

I also shop at the wholesale buying clubs. While they may be notorious for providing large quantities of junk foods, they are making great strides at offering more organic and additive free options. Many meats are now organic, so if you don't have a great local source for meats, that could be an option.

They also provide organic snack foods which are especially beneficial for school or picnic lunches and traveling. You can usually find frozen meals and fresh produce that are organic and/or additive free, and the cheese selection is often filled with raw milk cheeses and natural or organic cheeses. By buying these in bulk, the savings are significant.

When buying cheeses and other perishable items from these stores, I usually break the item up into usual size portions - 8 ounce blocks of cheese for example - and store the extra in the freezer in airtight packaging until I need it. That prevents the extra from going bad, ruining my savings.

Buying in bulk will require a little flexibility in your budget. Buying a year's worth of grain at once may be half of your usual budget for the whole grocery trip. But, you won't buy grain again for the year. You may need to spread out these larger purchases, or your budget may allow you to spend your annual grocery budget unevenly throughout the year. However you make it work, focus on prioritizing these savings. Because, as long as you stick to items you routinely use and don't go overboard, these deep savings will significantly reduce your annual grocery costs.

**Freezing Fresh Produce**

One of the most important steps when buying fresh produce in bulk is to freeze it correctly. I use this chart from the Colorado State University Extension Office:

Asparagus
Select young, tender stalks with compact tips. Remove or break off tough ends and scales. Wash thoroughly. Sort for size. Cut to fit containers or in 2-inch lengths. Blanch medium stalks 4 minutes in boiling water, 5 minutes in steam. Blanch large stalks 5 minutes in boiling water, 6 minutes in steam. Cool and drain dry. Pack without headspace, alternating tips and stem ends of spears.

Beans, green
Select young, tender stringless beans. Wash thoroughly, remove ends, sort for size. Cut into 1- to 2-inch pieces, leave whole, or slice into lengthwise strips. Water blanch 4 minutes. Chill and drain. Dry pack with headspace, or tray pack.

Beans, lima
Select well-filled pods containing green beans. Wash, shell and sort. Water blanch 3-5 minutes, depending on size. Cool and drain dry. Tray pack or dry pack with headspace.

Beans, green soybeans
Select firm, well-filled, bright green pods. Wash. Water blanch 6 minutes. Cool and drain. Squeeze soybeans out of pods. Dry pack with headspace, or tray pack.

Beets
Select beets 3 inches in diameter or less. Wash; sort for size. Remove tops, leaving 1/2-inch stems. Cook in boiling water until tender: 25-30 minutes for small beets, 45-50 minutes for medium-sized beets. Cool and drain; peel, slice or cube. Dry pack with headspace.

Broccoli
Select tender, dark green stalks. Wash; peel and trim stalks. To remove insects from heads, soak 30 minutes in a solution of 4 teaspoons of salt per gallon of water. Rinse and drain. Split lengthwise into pieces not more than 1 1/2 inches across. Blanch in steam 6 minutes or boiling water 4 minutes. Cool and drain. Dry or tray pack without headspace.

Brussels sprouts
Select green, firm and compact heads. Wash and trim. Soak in salt solution (see broccoli) 30 minutes to drive out insects. Rinse and drain. Water blanch 4-6 minutes depending on size of head. Cool and drain. Dry pack without headspace.

Cabbage
Wash. Trim coarse outer leaves of solid heads. Cut heads into medium or coarse shreds, thin wedges or separate into leaves. Water blanch 2 1/2 minutes. Cool and drain. Dry pack with headspace.

Carrots
Select tender, mild-flavored carrots. Remove tops; wash and peel. Leave whole if small; dice or slice larger carrots 1/4-inch thick. Water blanch whole carrots 6 minutes, diced or sliced carrots 3 minutes. Cool and drain. Dry pack with headspace.

Cauliflower
Choose firm, tender snow-white heads. Break or cut into pieces 1 inch across. Wash well. Soak 1/2 hour in salt brine (see broccoli) if needed to drive out insects. Rinse and drain. Blanch 4 minutes in boiling water containing 4 teaspoons salt per gallon of water. Cool and drain. Dry pack without headspace.

Corn, cut
Husk, remove silk, trim ends and wash. Water blanch 5 minutes. Cool and drain. Cut kernels from cob. Dry pack with headspace, or tray pack.

### Corn-on the-cob
Husk, remove silk, wash, sort for size. Water blanch small ears 8 minutes, medium ears 10 minutes and large ears 12 minutes. Cool and drain. Pack in plastic freezer bags without headspace.

### Eggplant
Peel, cut into slices 1/3-inch thick. To preserve color, drop pieces into a solution of 4 teaspoons salt per gallon of water. Water blanch 5 minutes in same proportions of salt and water. Cool and drain. Tray pack or dry pack in layers separated by sheets of locker paper.

### Greens
Wash young, tender leaves well. Remove tough stems and imperfect parts. Cut in pieces, if desired. Water blanch tender spinach leaves 2 1/2 minutes; beet greens, kale, chard, mustard greens, turnip and mature spinach leaves 3 minutes; and collard greens 4 minutes. Cool and drain. Dry pack with headspace.

### Herbs
Wash, drain, trim or chop. Tray freeze. Use in cooked dishes, as product becomes limp when thawed.

### Mushrooms
Select mushrooms free of spots or decay. Sort for size. Wash and drain. Trim off ends of stems. Slice or quarter mushrooms larger than 1 inch across. Dip mushrooms to be steam blanched for 5 minutes in solution of 1 teaspoon lemon juice or 1 1/2 teaspoons citric acid per pint of water. Steam whole mushrooms 6 minutes; quarters or slices 4-4 1/2 minutes. Cool and drain. Mushrooms also may be lightly sauteed in butter or margarine and cooled. Dry pack with headspace.

### Onions
Wash, peel and chop fully mature onions. Water blanch 2 1/2 minutes; cool and drain. Also may freeze without blanching. Tray pack or dry pack with headspace. Use in cooked products. Will keep 3-6 months.

Peas, green
Select bright green, plump, firm pods with sweet, tender peas. Shell. Water blanch 2 1/2 minutes. Cool and drain. Dry pack with headspace. Peas, sugar, or snow pod Wash, remove stems, blossom end and any strings. Leave whole. Water blanch 3 1/2 minutes. Cool and drain. Dry pack with headspace, or tray pack.

Peppers, green, sweet
Select firm, crisp, thick-walled peppers. Wash; cut out stems. Cut in half, remove seeds. Cut into strips or rings, if desired. Water blanch halves 4 minutes, slices 3 minutes for tighter packing and use in cooked dishes. Cool and drain. Freeze without blanching for use in salads and as garnishes. Dry pack blanched peppers with headspace. Tray or dry pack unblanched peppers without headspace.

Peppers, hot, condiment
Wash and stem peppers. Dry or tray pack in small containers without headspace.

Peppers, chili
Wash. Make a small slit in the side for steam to escape. Heat in 400-450 degree Farenheit oven 6-8 minutes or until skins blister. Cool in ice water for a crisp product. For a more thoroughly cooked product, wrap in a hot damp towel and allow to steam 15 minutes. Freeze without peeling or slit side, peel off skin and remove stem, seeds, membranes. Flatten to remove air, fold in half. Dry pack with waxed paper between single layers leaving headspace, or tray pack.

Pimentos
Wash. Roast in oven at 400 degrees Farenheit for 3-4 minutes. Rinse in cold water to remove charred skins. Drain. Dry pack with headspace, or tray pack.

Potatoes
Wash and peel; remove eyes, bruises, green spots. Cut in 1/4-1/2-inch cubes. Water blanch 4-6 minutes. Cool and dry pack with 1/2-inch headspace, or tray pack. For hash browns, cook in jackets until almost done. Peel and grate. Form in desired shapes. Pack and freeze. For French fries, peel and cut in thin strips. Rinse and dry. Fry in fat heated to 360 degrees Farenheit for 4 minutes or until golden. Drain and cool. Dry pack with headspace, or tray pack.

Pumpkins and winter squash (banana, butternut, buttercup)
Wash; cut into pieces and remove seeds. Cook pieces until soft in boiling water, steam, microwave oven, pressure cooker or 350-400 degree Farenheit oven (cut side down). Cool. Scoop out pulp; mash, blend or put through sieve. Chill thoroughly. Pack with headspace.

Rutabagas
Cut off tops of young, medium-sized rutabagas, wash and peel. Cut into cubes and water blanch 3 minutes. Cool, drain and dry pack with 1/2-inch headspace, or tray pack. For mashed rutabagas, cut into chunks and cook until tender in boiling water. Drain, mash, cool thoroughly and pack in containers with headspace.

Squash, summer (zucchini, yellow, white scallop)
Select young squash with small seeds and tender rind. Wash, cut in 1/2-inch slices. Water blanch 4 minutes. Cool and drain. Dry pack with headspace. Sweet potatoes Select medium to large mature sweet potatoes that have been air-dried (cured). Sort for size; wash. Cook until almost tender in water, steam, pressure cooker or oven. Cool at room temperature. Peel; cut in halves, slice, or mash. To prevent darkening, dip halves or slices in solution of either 1 tablespoon citric acid or 1/2 cup lemon juice per quart of water for 5 minutes. For mashed sweet potatoes, mix 2 tablespoons orange or lemon juice with each quart. Dry pack with headspace.

Tomatoes, juice
Wash, sort and trim firm tomatoes. Cut in quarters or eighths. Simmer 5-10 minutes. Press through sieve. Season with 1 teaspoon salt per quart of juice, if desired. Pour into containers, leaving 1 1/2-inch headspace.

Tomatoes, stewed
Wash ripe, blemish-free tomatoes. Scald 2-3 minutes to loosen skins; peel and core. Cut into pieces and freeze or simmer 10-20 minutes until tender. Cool and dry pack with 1/2-inch headspace.

Turnips; parsnips
Select tender, firm, mild-flavored small to medium turnips or parsnips. Wash, peel, cut into 1/2-inch cubes. Water blanch 3 minutes. Cool and drain. Dry pack with headspace.

## Tip Number Ten
## Farm to Table

While modern transportation methods have greatly improved public health by ensuring that a steady supply of fresh foods can be readily available to communities and towns when necessary, this long distance between the farm and table isn't as harmless to the grocery budget as we often like to think.

Costs set in place for groceries are dictated by the increasing cost of fuel for travel and by going rates for various food items. Due to these factors, they're pretty set throughout the year, even though different regions have different harvest sizes due to varying weather conditions. During times of threatened famine, this was a benefit. Now that we have more stable food production methods in advanced countries, there is a benefit to shortening this distance whenever possible.

We've already discussed the health benefits of locally produced food. By enabling produce to ripen on the vine, in the ground, or wherever it has been developing, we can obtain the most nutrient dense foods available.

However, by reducing the distance from farm to table, we can also significantly reduce the cost of our food as well. So healthier food for less than we'd pay for conventional food = win/win!

One of the easiest ways to save on food by getting them closer to home is to grow a potted herb garden in the kitchen. Fresh, organic herbs are usually several dollars at the grocery store and they never last long. However, a plant can be established for less than it costs to buy a small packet of herbs and will provide an endless supply of free fresh herbs for the kitchen!

In addition to providing free meal enhancements, the herbs are attractive decorations for the kitchen and have great aromas that eliminate the need for air freshener in the kitchen. Plus, they have great health benefits. Studies routinely show that herbs are some of the most concentrated sources of phytonutrients such as antioxidants. So keeping a basil or rosemary plant by the stove gives your meals a gourmet culinary twist plus a health boost. To top it off, most culinary herbs are very simple to grow and require little to no maintenance. So even if you don't have a green thumb, you shouldn't have any trouble getting a few culinary herbs established in your kitchen. For more tips, check out our book *The Kitchen Herbal*, which covers 18 culinary herbs, how to grow them, and how to use them.

Naturally, the next step for reducing the distance between the farm and table is to grow some of your own food in the backyard. This is often much easier than we believe it to be. Despite the countless sources for advice when it comes to gardening, little to no skill is actually required. Our ancestors managed to grow their own food for years and we can, too.

The key is to start small and be realistic. Begin with a container garden, a few pots with tomato plants or small berry bushes will do. Make sure to source your seeds or seedlings from suppliers that offer heirloom seeds to avoid GMOs and follow their instructions.

If you have kids, expand a little to a themed garden. Grow some basil, tomatoes, herbs and assorted veggies and call it a pizza garden. Form the plants into a circle pattern for even more fun.

If gardening isn't for you or you're already there, consider expanding outside of plant growth. Most modern cities now have provisions that allow small numbers of laying hens to be kept in the backyard, even in neighborhoods. These are relatively easy to keep and provide great experience with domestic animals - plus the fresh eggs make the additional work well worth it. And if you're getting eggs from local farmers, you usually save when you keep your own hens.

If you're ready to expand beyond laying hens, the options are limitless. Large scale gardens, goats, cows, etc, are all great ways to reduce the space between the farm and table, and usually provide great savings on healthier foods!

## Tip Number Eleven
## Doing it Myself

When evaluating the grocery list for excess and waste, it's easy to overlook many items that can be prepared at home - in seconds - for much less.

For example, when you begin eliminating salad dressings that are packed with additives, you may notice that the natural options are two to three times the price! And what's worse, these natural options still have added stabilizers, emulsifiers and "natural" additives! Why pay $4-$8 for something you can toss together at home in seconds? And if you have kids, this is a great project to assign to a budding chef or home cook.

Obviously making something at home means allocating additional time to the task. So it's important to make sure that the task and savings are worth the additional time. My criteria - it must result a substantial cost savings and/or a significant increase in nutrient content. It also must be relatively quick and easy to toss together at home - effortlessly. Your personal criteria may be different. If you have some additional leisure time and enjoy being in the kitchen, you may want to make more of these items, even if the cost savings is slight. Or you may not want to develop the skills necessary to make certain items at home. Either way, you can significantly reduce the grocery bill by looking through the list and choosing the items you want to make yourself at home. Here are a few of my homemade staples:

**Bars**

Breakfast bars are some of the most overpriced items at the grocery store, but are definitely handy on busier days!

**Cereal and Fruit Bars**

On the go breakfast foods were a great idea, but most contain those dreaded words: hydrogenated oils and high fructose corn syrup. Not to mention the wastefulness of the individual wrapping and unreasonable cost. Like most of our recipes, these are simple to make at home and provide beneficial fiber and B vitamins from the whole wheat, healthy proteins and fats from the nuts, butter and grains, and just the right blend of fats/carbohydrates/proteins to jump start your day!

1 cup (2 sticks) organic butter
1/3 cup honey
1/3 cup sucanat
1 1/2 cups whole wheat flour
1/2 cup almond meal (or almond flour or ground almonds)
2 cups oats
1 cup strawberry preserves / jam
1 teaspoon vanilla extract
1/2 teaspoon salt
1/2 teaspoon baking powder

Blend the butter and sweeteners. Combine with remaining ingredients. press 1/2 - 2/3 of the dough into a buttered square 8x8 pan. Spread the fruit on top, then press the remaining dough over the fruit. Bake at 350 for 25-30 minutes. For a thinner variety (like the store bought version) use a 9x13 pan and increase the fruit to 1 1/2 cups.

## Chocolate Chip Granola Bars

Granola bars have become the staple "go-to" food for traveling and long shopping trips. Yet, most granola bars are packed with hydrogenated oils, high fructose corn syrup and cheapened, artificial ingredients. These homemade treats are still sweet and dessert-like, but contain natural ingredients that our bodies recognize. The oats provide some whole grains, offsetting the sweetener content, and natural dark chocolate chips contain antioxidants! Adding walnuts or another healthy nut also contributes to the protein content and provides healthy fats that actually help our bodies lose weight! Better yet - these are simple to make and serve as a great recipe for young girls learning to use the kitchen.

4 cups oats
1/2 cup dark chocolate chips (natural, with cocoa butter, not hydrogenated oils)
2/3 cup brown rice syrup (honey or a blend of agave nectar and a sugar syrup can also be used)
1/3 cup sucanat
3 Tablespoons organic butter
2 teaspoons vanilla extract (fair trade, organic)
1 teaspoon salt
1 cup chopped nuts (optional)

Preheat the oven to 350 degrees. Butter a 9x9 inch baking pan; set aside. Spread the oats and nuts over a large baking sheet and toast in preheated oven for 10-12 minutes, stirring every 2-3 minutes. Set aside to cool. In a small saucepan, mix the sweeteners together over low heat until the sucanat dissolves and the two are thoroughly blended. Set aside to cool. Once cooled, toss everything together in a large bowl, stir to combine thoroughly. Press mixture into the prepared pan and bake for 25-30 minutes. When cooled, cut into 12 large or 16 regular sized bars.

## Condiments

Most condiments contain additives and preservatives that we try to avoid. Finding freshly produced options usually means spending much more. Here are a few of our favorites that I can throw together relatively quickly.

## BBQ Sauce

A good jar of bbq sauce makes a quick weeknight meal. Add some chicken, corn and potatoes and you're all set. The recipe makes quite a bit, so you only have to make it once for 2 meals. Store the leftover sauce in the fridge and use within 2-3 weeks. (This makes a sweet, creamy sauce. For a traditional vinegar based sauce, see below.)

1 T sunflower oil
1 T onion powder (or 1/2 onion, minced)
1 clove garlic, minced
1 1/2 cup organic ketchup
1/4 cup molasses
1 T sucanat
1 t red pepper flakes, crushed
2 T mustard
1 T worcestershire sauce
Juice of 1 lemon
Salt and pepper, to taste

Warm the oil in a saucepan over medium heat. Add the onions and garlic. Simmer for 2-3 minutes, then add the remaining ingredients. Simmer 1-2 additional minutes. Enjoy!

**Stir Fry Sauce**

This quick and easy sauce does require some stove time, but makes a quick and easy dinner to prepare later. Toss some chopped veggies (broccoli, asparagus, carrots, onions, zucchini, peppers, squash, eggplant, or anything you have on hand) into a pan with some of this sauce. Add some chicken (optional) and cook thoroughly for a fast weeknight favorite. Scoop onto brown rice for a complete meal.

1/3 cup sesame oil
1/4 cup soy sauce
1-2 cloves garlic
2 T chopped ginger
1 teaspoon crushed red pepper
1 T cornstarch
1/4 cup chicken stock

Combine the garlic, ginger and 2 T of the sesame oil in a saucepan over medium heat. Cook until the herbs are aromatic. Remove from heat. Add the cornstarch and chicken stock. Combine until thickened. Add remaining ingredients. Cool. Bottle. Store in the fridge 3-4 weeks.

## Extracts

Avoiding artificial flavorings is essential for the real foods diet, but the natural extracts are much more expensive than the artificial versions - sometimes three to four times the cost. It's easy to make your own and these make great gifts as well!

These recipes do include the use of vodka as most store bought flavoring extracts rely upon an alcohol to preserve the contents. This enables the extract to have a shelf life of 18-24 months.

## Vanilla Extract

2 vanilla beans
A tall bottle
1/2 cup vodka or other edible alcohol
3 T distilled water

Cut the bean in half lengthwise. Place the bean in the bottle. Add the alcohol. Add the water.

Cap and leave in a cabinet for 3-4 weeks until dark and aromatic. You can then remove the beans and strain the seeds or remove only the beans and leave the seeds for your baked goods.

Use as directed in your favorite recipe.

## Peppermint Extract

1/4 ounce dried mint leaves
A tall bottle
1/2 cup vodka or other edible alcohol
3 T distilled water

Place all of the ingredients in the bottle. Cap and let sit 3-4 weeks or until extract is colorful and aromatic. Strain and use in any recipe.

Variations: For orange, lemon or other extracts, substitute about 1/4 cup of dried herb or fruit peel for the peppermint leaves in the above recipe. Strain and use the extract as directed in your favorite recipes.

## Salad Dressings

These must haves are also usually packed with additives and fillers, and obtaining a healthier option usually doubles, if not triples the price. Additionally, they rarely last long in the fridge, so the wasted extra dressing adds even more to the overall grocery bill. These small batch recipes are perfect for quickly preparing your favorite dressing and can be halved if you don't plan on using it all before it goes bad.

## Ranch

A classic ranch dressing has multiple uses. Top a bowl of greens with this creamy sauce for a healthy but filling meal or use to dip fresh veggies. Natural ranch dressings are often pricey, but don't take long to make at home. (You can use fresh or dried herbs in this recipe. For fresh herbs, double the amount. For dried, stick to the same measurements.)

1/2 cup mayonnaise
1/2 cup sour cream
1/2 cup buttermilk
1/2 cup Greek yogurt
1 T dill
1 T chives
1 T parsley
1 clove chopped garlic
2 t fresh lemon juice

Combine well. Store in the fridge for up to 3-4 weeks.

**Blue Cheese**

This classic recipe is also a must have in the home. Use it as a healthier alternative for junk foods, as a salad dressing or on top of a wedge of iceberg.

1 cup sour cream
1/2 cup mayonnaise
1/2 cup buttermilk
2 T rice wine vinegar
1 T chopped chives
1 t salt
1/2 t pepper
4 ounces good quality blue cheese

Combine well in a bowl. For a creamy dip, pulse in a food processor. For a chunkier dip, simply mix with a spoon. Store in the fridge for 3-4 weeks.

**Salsas**

Store-bought salsas might not be the most expensive condiments on the shelf, but they're not nearly as tasty as a homemade version and during the summer when these vegetables are in season, the homemade option makes a big difference in cost.

**Homemade Salsa**

4 cups chopped fresh tomatoes
1/4 cup chopped green onions
1/2 cup chopped fresh cilantro
3 T pureed garlic
1 T chopped fresh oregano
2 T chopped fresh peppers (as hot as you like it)
1 each red, yellow green pepper, chopped
2 T oil
1/4 cup fresh lemon juice
salt and pepper to taste

Stir all ingredients together in a bowl. Let chill overnight for the flavors to mellow.

## Stocks

Chicken, beef and vegetable stocks are healthy additions to any meal. Not only do they enhance the flavor, they dramatically increase the nutrient content. However, the store bought options are usually either packed with MSG or other additives or very expensive. And they rarely can compare to the flavor of a homemade stock., which is surprisingly easy to make.

## Chicken Stock

1 chicken carcass
6-8 cups water
2 carrots, chopped
1 medium onion, chopped
2 stalks of celery, chopped
Handful of various herbs

Toss everything together in a large stockpot. Bring to a simmer. Cover. Simmer for 4-8 hours. If water levels drop, add more water until the levels are high enough to cover the carcass.

After simmering, let cool. Strain out the vegetables and chicken bits. Store in the fridge for up to 3-5 days or freeze for later use.

For beef stock, substitute beef bones and add 1/4 cup tomato paste. For veggie stock, omit the bones.

**Vinaigrettes**

These healthy kitchen staples are usually not only pricey but packed with additives to maintain texture and color. However, they can be tossed together in seconds at home with ingredients you probably already keep on hand. These homemade creations are simple to make, are much healthier than the additive laden store bought versions, and are made for a fraction of the cost.

Here's a simple recipe for a basic vinaigrette. Customize it by adding herbs, cheeses, nuts or even dried fruit. You can also play around with the types of oil and vinegar to make gourmet vinaigrettes that are perfectly suited to your favorite greens.

This makes an apple-mustard vinaigrette. You can add tiny chopped apples for more apple flavor. Omitting the mustard is an option, but the vinaigrette will separate much sooner.

1/2 cup olive oil (quality is important here)
3 tablespoons raw apple cider vinegar
2 teaspoons dijon mustard (this acts as an emulsifier, keeping your vinaigrette from separating as rapidly)
1/2 teaspoon salt
dash fresh black pepper

Combine everything in a jar. Stir rapidly with a fork and serve. The mustard (which can be omitted if you prefer) will help keep it together for a couple of hours, but it will need to be stirred again when you use if later. It can be stored in the fridge for 1-2 weeks on average, depending on the added ingredients you use.

Olive oil is a heart healthy monounsaturated fat that provides numerous antioxidants and phytonutrients - chemicals that protect against cancer and promote health! It helps to support the liver in its daily detoxification process, balances blood sugar and contributes to weight control. Vinegar is a medicinal agent that serves as a digestive aid - ensuring that maximum nutrient absorption from your healthy meals. It also helps to strengthen the liver and helps to reduce depression. Unfiltered and traditionally fermented vinegars are ideal, as the white distilled vinegar can leach minerals from the body, is often made from synthetic ingredients and does not provide the same benefits.

**Tip:** I store all of my homemade marinates, sauces and dressings in regular glass canning jars. These jars have many advantages over the costly storage containers available:
- They are glass, not metal or plastic, so I don't have to worry about chemicals leeching into my acidic products.
- They are available for about $8 per dozen at most grocers, making them extremely cost efficient.
- They are dishwasher safe - so quick and easy clean up when I'm done!
- They come with secure lids - just a quick shake and they are ready to pour!
- They are versatile - I can use them for numerous homemade treats.

## Tip Number Twelve
## Save it for Later

So, I've mentioned that we always try to avoid having leftovers. However, that doesn't mean that we miss out on the quick dinnertime meals that can be enjoyed by serving leftovers; I frequently intentionally cook extra to put away for later. I just don't call them leftovers.

The trick to healthy eating is to make sure that you're always prepared for last minute needs. An extra errand throughout the day that leaves no time for dinner. Tasks that take longer than we had planned. Last minute guests. We've all experienced those situations where we're basically stuck. There's not the hour or so necessary to prepare a proper meal, so we reluctantly call for pizza delivery or take other shortcuts because *something* is better than nothing.

Preparing a few additional meals ahead of time can eliminate the situations that dictate compromises in my mealtime standards. When I'm making something like lasagna, it's just as easy to make a second one. Then I toss the extra in the freezer and it's ready when I need it. I can make extra pizza dough, cooked peas or beans, and many other items that usually require lengthy preparation times at once, then store them in the freezer until I need them.

**Things that freeze well:**

Baked pasta dishes such as ziti or lasagna
Black eyed peas
Cooked beans - any kind (freeze in the liquid)
Creamed corn
Risotto
Polenta
Pureed foods

**Foods to prepare ahead of time:**

Chicken (I cook a whole bird then freeze the shredded meat)
Chopped veggies (chop and freeze)
Hard boiled eggs (store in the fridge for 7-10 days)
Salad Dressings
Sauces

**Frozen lasagna** is a go-to quick dinner option that has potential as a health food, but rarely comes close to being healthy OR flavorful in its many frozen varieties. This homemade version takes a day's worth of work and spreads it out for those busier days when just sitting down seems to be unthinkable. Serve with a fast green salad topped with the homemade vinaigrette you have stored in the fridge and some quick garlic bread and a full meal is ready to go in minutes.

9 eggs
3 pounds dried lasagna sheets
5 ten ounce packages frozen spinach, thawed and drained
2 cups shredded parmesan cheese
6 cups shredded mozzarella cheese
3 pounds ricotta cheese
5 cups tomato-basil sauce
8 cups milk
1 cup whole wheat flour
3/4 cup organic butter

optional: 1-2 pounds grass fed, hormone and antibiotic free ground beef

Begin by making a classic white sauce. In a medium saucepan, combine the butter with the flour. Whisk together as the butter melts. When smooth, add the milk, slowly, whisking continually until it is all blended. Simmer until the sauce has thickened, about 12 minutes. Remove from heat.

If using the beef, brown with 2-3 crushed cloves of garlic and 1/2 onion, chopped. Set aside to cool. Cook the pasta sheets until softened but still firm.

Mix the ricotta and eggs in another bowl. Add the tomato basil sauce to the white sauce. There should now be a bowl of sauce, a bowl of ricotta/egg mixture, a bowl of beef, a bowl of spinach, and bowls of each of the remaining cheeses.

Take three 9x13 pans - ensuring that at least 2 of them are freezer/oven safe. Spread the sauce over the bottom of each pan. Top with a layer of lasagna sheets. Add the remaining ingredients in the following order: all of the ricotta, all of the spinach, pasta, beef (all of it - if using), 1/2 the mozzarella, sauce, pasta, sauce, all remaining cheese.

Cover two of the freezer safe pans securely and freeze for up to 8 weeks. Bake the other pan at 375 for 45 minutes. Drizzle with 3 tablespoons olive oil while still hot. to bake the frozen lasagna, place in a 400 degree oven and bake for 45-60 minutes, drizzling with the oil when finished.

## Homemade Pizzas (dough recipe makes 12 crusts)

Frozen pizzas are not only convenient, they can be a great at-home healthy "fast food" for busy days. This recipe makes 12 small sized pizza crusts - perfect for small families OR big families with a variety of palates.

12 cups whole wheat flour
3 packets baker's yeast (for naturally leavened dough, use 1 cup sourdough starter and increase the rising time by 1 hour)
1/4 cup olive oil
1 T salt
2 T honey
6 cups water (give or take 1/2 cup, depending on the humidity)

Combine everything in a large bowl. If using a stand mixer, mix in 2 batches with the dough hook then hand knead it all together. Otherwise, hand knead the dough until it is pliable and smooth. Leave lightly covered to rise 1-2 hours or until doubled. Divide the dough into 12 equal sized balls. Let rest 10 minutes then flatten to form 8 inch discs. If using right away, glaze with olive oil and place your desired toppings.

Bake at 500 degrees for 8-10 minutes until the crust is golden brown and the cheese is bubbly. With the remaining discs, bake at 500 for 3-5 minutes until the dough is cooked but not browned. Remove and allow to cool. Freeze 2-3 hours, then wrap tightly in plastic wrap. Place back in the freezer until ready to use (up to 2-3 months) To use, remove and allow to thaw partially - about 20 minutes. Apply toppings and bake at 500 degrees until browned.

## Tip Number Thirteen
## Allergies and Sensitivities

One of the biggest constraints on a real foods budget is working with food allergies and sensitivities, which are growing in number among modern populations. These foods, while absolutely necessary, are often very expensive and can quickly eat up the budget, especially if it's already tight.

How to cope? Just about all of the tips listed previously in this book apply to those with food sensitivities and allergies. Avoid processed foods, make things from scratch when possible, and look for better deals than what's available at the grocery store. Here's another: skip the allergen friendly food.

Some of the most processed foods available in a conventional grocery store are the allergy-friendly foods marketed to individuals such as yourselves. These foods are usually produced with highly refined grains, excessive sweeteners and/or artificial substitutes for the allergen.

For example, gluten free products frequently cost 2-4 times more than their gluten containing counterparts, but their ingredient list is packed with refined, processed, and additive based ingredients. These ingredients are not doing anything to help repair the damage that gluten has been causing the individual for months or years, and can even contribute to further inflammation.

What's more, these products can be prepared at home for much less, in a short amount of time, with nutrient dense ingredients that promote healing. In the Guide to Bread: Unlocking the Mysteries of Grains, Gluten and Yeast, I cover how easy it is to make a healthy, nourishing, gluten free bread that has a crust and crumb similar to gluten containing breads.

Likewise, dairy free cheeses and frozen foods are similarly refined and processed, offering no real benefit. While they can't generally be produced at home, they usually don't offer the cheese-like taste and texture that a dairy free individual is longing for. And they're very expensive. So, those with allergies are stuck paying a fortune for a product that doesn't have much to offer.

As an example, I've included some of my favorite allergen free recipes over the next couple of pages.

**Dairy Free Strawberry Lemon Cheesecake**

3 cups cashews
2/3 cup fresh lemon juice
2/3 cup honey
1 cup coconut oil
1/2 cup crushed strawberries
1 teaspoon salt
1 tablespoon vanilla extract

Pulse all ingredients (except the berries) together in a blender on medium to high for 30-34 seconds or until finely combined.

Pour into a graham cracker crust. Add the strawberries and swirl the red berries around the yellow filling with a knife. Set in the fridge until firm - about 24 hours. Serve with additional fresh berries. Enjoy!

**My Favorite GF Cookies**

These are packed with nutrients and yummy bits of chocolate. And the best part is that nobody will ever guess that they're gluten free!

1 1/2 cup almond flour
1 cup oats
1/2 cup sorghum flour
1/4 cup cornstarch
1/2 t baking soda
1 1 baking powder
1/2 cup rolled oats
1/2 cup walnuts
1 cup organic candy coated chocolate (I use Sunspire brand)

Combine everything together in a bowl. Scoop into 1 tablespoon chunks on a parchment lined cookie sheet and bake at 350 degrees until golden brown - about 10-12 minutes.

** For nut allergies, substitute 2/3 cup flaxseed meal combined with 2/3 cup garbanzo bean flour for the almond meal and 1/2 cup sunflower seeds for the walnuts.**

## Ice Cream Sandwiches, Gluten Free

My motto is that no real food is bad, they have just been prepared with terrible recipes. Many favorite junk foods could actually be a great part of a real foods diet, as long as they are prepared correctly and kept in moderation. Ice cream and ice cream sandwiches are a great example of this. Any natural chocolate cookie can be used for a traditional sandwich. Below is a gluten free option for children that do not need to consume gluten. These ice cream sandwiches are so good that even guests that are not on a gluten free diet will love them!

>   1/2 cup buckwheat flour
>   1/4 cup cornstarch
>   1 T garbanzo bean flour
>   1/4 cup cocoa powder
>   1 stick butter
>   1/4 cup chocolate chips
>   1 cup sucanat
>   1/4 cup agave nectar
>   1 t salt
>   3 eggs
>   2 t vanilla extract

Over low heat, melt the butter and chocolate chips together. Remove from heat and add the sugar, salt, eggs and vanilla. When combined, add the remaining dry ingredients. Mixture will be resemble brownie batter. Spread in a thin layer onto a lined cookie sheet. Bake at 350 for 12-15 minutes or until a toothpick comes clean. While still warm, pierce with a fork and score into squares (or cut into circles using a ice cream sandwich mold). When cooled, pack a scoop of softened ice cream in between 2 cookies and place in the freezer to firm. Makes 6-12 sandwiches, depending on size of squares.

## Tip Number Fourteen
## Avoiding Burnout

One key to ensuring that real foods fit into a realistic budget is to avoid burnout. We've all seen it, if not experienced it - the grocery cart is packed with healthy foods and the kitchen is fully stocked. Yet, the standard has been set so high that it's difficult to maintain.

When the family won't eat the foods we've purchased, we're not saving money on anything; we're wasting money on food that is tossed. It doesn't matter if the pantry is filled with real foods. When the foods aren't what they want and we order pizza instead, we pay for dinner twice.

So, the key to making the real foods budget work is to make sure that the standards we want to implement in our families are realistic and match where we are on the journey to natural health.

This doesn't mean giving up; it means taking the time for the new habits to be fully adapted by the family, one at a time, until the whole diet has converted to real foods. Here are a few tips from my book The Vintage Remedies Guide to Real Food:

**Start Small**

Rome wasn't built in a day, and anything worth working for will take some time to get right. When people come to learn about the major concerns with the typical food system, they tell me about heading to the grocery store to find it is no longer filled with cereal, snacks and drinks. Instead, they can find nothing but high fructose corn syrup, hydrogenated oils and artificial colors! Where did the food go? Often leaving frustrated after an hour or two of finding nothing suitable for the family to eat, the path to a healthier diet reaches its first main roadblock, and *overwhelmed* becomes an understatement.

This feeling is completely understandable, and quite common. The desire to change has set in, but the taste buds, eating habits and cooking habits have yet to catch up. Instead of trying to change everything right out of the gate, I recommend prioritizing the changes and working on them one or two at a time. Choose what affects your family the most, whether it be high fructose corn syrup, conventional meats, preservatives or hydrogenated oils. Start there, master the change, then work towards the next goal.

This allows the family to slowly adjust to the new habit, and removes much of the guilt and frustration that occurs with an overnight change in the pantry. Sure, it allows certain habits to continue longer than you may want them to, but the changes you make one at a time are longer lasting and more permanent than overnight makeovers, which are generally met with resistance. I recommend picking a goal that is easy to meet, to get some momentum going for the next one. It is easier to keep it going than to start and stop in the manner of yo-yo dieting.

Additionally, overnight changes are not healthy for the diet. Learning to adapt to increased fiber intake from whole grains or more vegetables takes some time for the body. Many people find that changes that occur too quickly generally lead to an overall feeling of sluggishness, fatigue and other related problems during the first few weeks, as the body adjusts and purges itself of some of the toxins that have been built up over the years. While this is necessarily unhealthy, it can be a deterrent to further change and is often frustrating to deal with. One common example of this is the caffeine headache so commonly associated with "cold turkey" quitting. Additionally, changes to real foods often result in weight loss, something that should also happen gradually to prevent many serious health concerns as the body changes too quickly. The best way to avoid these risks and concerns is to make changes slowly and gradually, allowing the body to adapt fully before moving on.

**Set Attainable Goals**

Even with the one step at a time approach, if the first step is to cut out the family's favorite dish, replacing it with something dramatically different, the challenge may prove to be too much. Likewise, if you allow yourself just one week to meet a new goal before moving on to the next, you could be setting yourself up for failure. Instead, be realistic with the goals and deadlines you give yourself and your family.

Setting attainable goals is the best way to ensure the plan is workable and allows the maximum opportunity to meet the goals, enjoying the benefits of a healthier diet, rather than the stress of changing too quickly. Meals should be enjoyable, not stressful and with healthy, real foods, there is no reason to make something challenging or difficult when it should be fun and inviting.

## Slow and Steady Wins the Race

I have found that the best way to meet each goal is to work gradually. Instead of dumping the bleached white bread and baking a batch of whole wheat sourdough bread, which most families immediately reject, a gradual introduction to the nutty, tangy flavor of whole wheat sourdough can be slowly increased until they find they actually prefer the taste.

For flour, try substituting 10% of the white flour with whole wheat. Chances are, nobody will even notice. Stick with this for a few days, then increase it to 20%. A few days later, try 30%, then 40% then half. Gradually, the whole wheat flour will completely replace the white flour; meanwhile the family has had the time to adjust to the difference in taste. When this happens, they will suddenly notice that a slice of bread baked with refined, white flour has a gummy, bland taste, and lifelong habits will have been established.

For breads, baking at home may be too much of a task to begin with, and if that is the case, consider looking for a local bakery that bakes real bread. I always ask to see the ingredient list and look for the word "yeast." If it is not there, they use a natural starter, and the bread is going to be so much better than most (sometimes all) of what is available at a grocery store.

Most healthy eating habits lend themselves well to baby steps. If the children love sodas, start changing to organic sodas, moving to fruit juice based carbonated drinks, then to homemade fizzy juice drinks from Chapter Ten for parties and special celebrations.

## Quality Over Quantity

Another benefit to the slow and steady approach is that it allows time to focus on quality, not quantity. Anyone can spend a fortune purchasing new ingredients and home appliances and start baking whole wheat snacks, homemade breads and real foods tomorrow, but without the benefit of experience, the results will be less than stellar. Learning how to prepare grass fed meats takes some time, as they cook differently than conventional meats. Whole grains don't work in every recipe and many additional minor changes will need to be made.

By mastering each skill before moving on, the quality of your homemade goods will be unbeatable. Any home cook can verify that the first homemade loaf of bread was great, but nothing like the 50th. As each loaf is prepared, the baker learns how the dough should feel, how weather affects the dough, how to tweak things a touch to perfect the recipe and how to bake it just the right way. The same is true for using new flours, new kitchen tools, new types of meat and new oils and fats.

Real foods are not only superior nutritionally, but also in taste and sustainability. Unfortunately, many well intended health food junkies have introduced some sub par products, leading many to believe that healthy foods are the opposite of delicious foods! The reality is that everything that makes a food healthy also makes it delicious. Gourmet chefs will be the first to choose real oils and fats over hydrogenated counterfeits. Processed foods were not introduced to the market for their superior taste and flavor, but as a way to cut corners, which they have done in price, taste, and appearance.

## Tip Number Fifteen
## Quick and Easy Standbys

Finally, the best tip I have is to always have an assortment of family favorites that you can prepare quickly and easily. Bonus points if an older child or other family member can also prepare this meal at the spur of the moment. This prevents last minute pizza delivery calls and trips to the drive through because you have a couple of real foods based meals ready to go at a moments notice.

I've included some of my family's favorites over the next few pages. They can easily be adapted to accommodate personal taste preferences and food allergies by eliminating or substituting allergen free ingredients. Enjoy!

## Lemony Fish with Parmesan Risotto

This is comfort cooking at its best. The slightly tangy flavor of the dill and lemon against the fish blends perfectly with the warm risotto. Better yet, the fish provide healthy omega 3 oils, which our bodies are usually lacking, but absolutely need, and the risotto is a creamy yet healthy dish with just a little bit of heart healthy fats. Serve with a green salad and some homemade bread for a more elaborate fare, or leave it as is for a quick weeknight dinner.

6 filets cod
3-4 tablespoons olive oil
1/2 cup flour
1 teaspoon salt
dash pepper
dash dill

Mix the flour and herbs together in a shallow bowl. Set aside. In a frying pan, heat the oil over medium high heat. Dredge the fish filets through the flour and cook 2-4 minutes on each side or until the fish is done. (Thicker cuts will require more cooking time.) Remove from the pan and garnish with fresh lemon juice and a lemon wedge.

1 cup risotto rice
4 cups chicken or veggie stock
1 teaspoon salt
2 cloves minced garlic
1 tablespoon olive oil

Heat the olive oil over medium heat. Add the garlic and let cook for 1-2 minutes, then add the dried rice. Add just enough stock to cover the rice and let simmer, stirring occasionally. Keep an eye on it and add more stock as needed, but only enough to cover the rice. When the rice is tender and most (or all) of the stock has been absorbed, remove from heat. It should be creamy and tender. Add 1/3 cup shredded parmesan. Serve hot.

**Pomegranate Chicken with Mandarin
served with garlic green beans**

Nothing makes an ordinary main course spectacular like a rich flavorful sauce. Yet, many commercial sauces rely on sweeteners to make up for a lack of flavor. A good sauce should be savory with deep flavors, not sweet and bland. Not only is this sauce amazingly delicious, it is simple to put together and a fraction of the cost of store bought / ready made sauces.

4 free range chicken breasts
2 mandarins, chopped
juice of 3 mandarins
1/4 cup pomegranate juice
1 T each butter and flour

Grill the chicken on an outdoor grill. Sprinkle with salt and pepper prior to grilling if desired. Take the mandarins, both fruit juices, butter and flour and mix together on the stovetop to make a smooth sauce. Add salt and pepper if desired. Spoon over grilled chicken and garnish with mandarin wedges.

For the beans: Pour 2-3 tablespoons of olive oil into a pan over medium heat. When hot, add 1 pound green beans and 2 minced garlic cloves. Sprinkle with sea salt and saute until tender but still firm. Serve immediately.

**Cilantro Lime Chicken Wraps**

This is a fun summery dish; I like to make it when we have company because it is easy to double or triple the recipe to feed a crowd. Served with fresh lime garnishes, homemade salsa and chips, this easy to prepare dish is transformed into an impressive spread.

4 limes
1 onion, diced
2 T honey
1/4 cup cilantro leaves
2 t minced garlic
4 free range chicken breasts (cutlets are ideal) 10 tortillas
1 cup shredded lettuce
1 cup shredded cheese (white cheddar is good) salsa (recipe above)
Zest and juice 3 of the limes; thinly slice the fourth.

In a bowl, combine the zest and juice with the honey, onion, garlic and cilantro. Reserve 2 T of the mixture. Grill the chicken, brushing the remaining lime mixture over the top. In a bowl, tear the chicken into small pieces and add the remaining lime mixture. Fill a tortilla with chicken, lettuce and cheese. Top with salsa. Serve garnished with additional salsa, sliced limes and crisp corn chips. Serves 5

**Pan Seared Sole with Chili Lime Butter**

1/2 stick unsalted butter, softened
1 T finely chopped shallot
1 t lime zest
2 t lime juice
1 t red pepper flakes
1/2 t salt

Mix ingredients together and set aside. This is the butter we will use to garnish the fish.

Sprinkle 4 filets with salt. Heat 1 T olive oil in a shallow pan over medium high heat. Two at a time, cook the fish in the heated oil 4-6 minutes until golden, turning halfway through. Remove to a serving dish and garnish with the lime butter and slices of fresh lime if desired.

**Tri Color Orzo**

Orzo is nothing more than a small, rice shaped pasta. The colors come from vegetable extracts, making it naturally kid friendly and healthy! This dish is a standby in our home. It needs to spend some time in the fridge for the flavors to blend, which makes it a perfect make ahead dish for busy evenings. It is best served chilled, but can also be served at room temperature and can be prepared up to 2 days in advance! For picky eaters, feel free to substitute any of the ingredients for those that are more familiar and comfortable.

> 1 pound tri color orzo
> 1/4 cup sun dried tomatoes, drained
> 1/2 cup Kalamata olives
> 8-10 artichoke hearts, drained
> 1/2 cup Italian herbed vinaigrette
> 1/4 cup shredded hard Italian cheese such as Parmesan
> 2-3 T pine nuts

Cook pasta according to package directions. (Do not overcook!) Rinse well with cool water. Stir in the vinaigrette, olives, tomatoes and artichokes. Chill, covered, for 2-4 hours. Remove and top with the cheese and nuts before serving.

Note: This dish can easily become a gluten free meal by substituting equal amounts of cooked quinoa for the orzo. Make sure the vinaigrette is gluten free!

## Arugula and Chevre Penne

Arugula is a green vegetable in the broccoli family. Adding it to a pasta dish elevates it from simple to gourmet, and the flavor in this recipe can't be beat! The cheese adds protein in an easy to digest form, and the tomatoes and greens provide an assortment of vitamins, minerals and phytonutrients.

6 ounces chevre, crumbled (goat cheese)
2 cups arugula, chopped
2/3 cup sun dried tomatoes in olive oil
2 t garlic paste (or minced garlic)
dash salt and pepper

Cook 1/2 pound of whole wheat penne pasta according to package directions. Drain and toss with the crumbled cheese, arugula, garlic and tomatoes. Add salt and pepper to taste and serve in 2 warm pasta dishes with crusty bread.

Note: This can easily become a gluten free meal by using gluten free pasta.

**Moroccan Lentil Soup**

2 chopped onions
1 t pureed garlic
1 cup red lentils
1 pound cooked chickpeas
1 15 ounce can diced tomatoes
1 cup sliced carrots
1/2 cup chopped celery
1.5 t ground cardamom
1/2 t cayenne pepper
1/2 t cumin

Add all the ingredients to a large stockpot and simmer for 2 hours with 5 cups of water. Add up to 1.5 more cups of water, if needed. Serve hot with bread.

## Dijon Maple Salmon

Maple syrup is gathered from the maple tree. When dried, it becomes maple sugar, which can be used in place of white sugar in recipes. Approximately forty gallons of sap are reduced to make one gallon of maple syrup. Maple syrup is a healthier choice than white sugar as it contains less sucrose. It still is processed quickly like other sugars, so it should be consumed in moderation. One caution with maple syrup is the lead seams in the metal cans some producers store the syrup in. Canadian maple syrup and certified organic syrup can be considered safe and lead free.

In addition to desserts, maple syrup can add a sweet glaze to vegetables or even main dishes, like in this Dijon Maple Glazed Salmon.

4 wild salmon filets
1/2 cup organic butter
1/2 cup maple syrup
1/4 cup Dijon mustard

Mix the mustard, butter and syrup together. Brush the salmon with this glaze while cooking over high heat until flaky and tender.

**Herb Shirred Eggs**

These are quick and easy, yet provide a fun alternative to the typical "scrambled or fried" routine. Don't worry about eggs and cholesterol - studies show that fresh eggs from healthy chickens don't increase cholesterol as a natural component within the eggs also works to decrease cholesterol! Eggs are fantastic foods, providing numerous useful ingredients, and the herbs serve as flavorful and potent antioxidants.

6 eggs
1/4 cup panko breadcrumbs (or fresh homemade breadcrumbs)
1/4 cup cheese (cheddar is great here, but mild cheeses are good as well)
1 teaspoon of each: dried parsley, dried rosemary, dried thyme
salt and pepper to taste

Crack each egg into a small ramekin. (Alternatively, place all eggs in a single small baking dish) In a small bowl, combine the remaining ingredients. Place 1 tablespoon of the topping mixture onto the raw egg and bake at 400 degrees for 6-8 minutes or until the egg is firm. Serve hot.

## Grilled Artichokes with Asparagus

Artichokes are important members of the thistle family and could be considered the whole foods version of milk thistle, an important liver supportive herb. While the mechanisms of action are different in the two plants, due to varying chemical constituents, both are valuable for assisting in the natural cleansing process. This makes a great dinner for cleansing programs but is also yummy enough to enjoy anytime.

4 large artichokes, rinsed well
3 T salt
2 lemons, sliced
2 cloves chopped garlic
olive oil
chopped fresh parsley

Remove the top of the artichokes and trim the leaves. Rub the cut sides with slices of lemon. Fill a large pot with water, the salt and the lemons and bring to a boil. Add the artichokes and simmer about 15-20 minutes until tender. (Note: to steam or otherwise prepare artichokes in water would take approx. 45 min to an hour. This step is just to prepare the artichokes for grilling.)

When the artichokes cool, cut in half, removing the purple insides and choke. Sprinkle salt, some pepper and the garlic over the artichoke halves then drizzle with olive oil. Place over a grill pan on the stove (or an outdoor grill) over high heat. Grill until the edges begin to blacken - about 5-7 minutes. Serve hot with a buttery garlic dipping sauce.

For the asparagus, rinse and trim the spears. Use the same garlic / salt / pepper preparation treatment mentioned above and place in the grill pan until just tender - about 3-5 minutes.

## Quinoa Primavera w/ Arugula Salad

One of my favorite ways to enjoy quinoa is as a vegetarian main dish as a substitute for pasta. Quinoa is gluten free, so this is also a great meal for anyone with celiac or gluten intolerance - a growing number of individuals! Unlike many wheat substitutes, quinoa is actually nutritionally superior to wheat - whereas many gluten free flours offer poor nutritional profiles. And the flavor is easily adaptable, allowing the main flavors to take center stage.

3 carrots, sliced
2 zucchini, cut into strips
1 onion, chopped
1 cup green peas
1/2 cup sun dried tomatoes, packed in olive oil
1/2 cup grated parmesan cheese
1/4 cup olive oil
2 cups quinoa (brown is easy to find but red is also fun and colorful!)

On a large baking sheet, place the carrots, zucchini and onions. Bake at 400 degrees until tender, about 15 minutes. While that is cooking, prepare the quinoa according to package directions, which should take between 15 and 20 minutes. Add the green peas during the last 5 minutes. Toss with the cooked vegetables, the olive oil and the cheese. Season with salt and pepper.

For the arugula salad, toss 2 cups arugula with 8-10 (halved) cherry tomatoes. Add a homemade vinaigrette, preferably a lemon based creation, and top with some additional parmesan cheese and crispy homemade croutons.

**Berry Sorbet**

This is not technically a sorbet, but the quick shortcut makes a sorbet - like treat and can be prepared in minutes! Berries provide potent cleansing antioxidants, fiber and plenty of wonderful phytonutrients.

1 cup each: frozen blueberries, strawberries, raspberries 1/2 cup white grape juice

Place into a food processor and pulse until nearly smooth. Serve slightly softened or place in the freezer up to 2 weeks. Scoop into a bowl and serve with fresh berries.

## Maple Bleu Cheese Salad

2 cups red romaine leaves
2 cups green romaine leaves
1/2 cup sliced red onion
1 green apple, chopped
2 stalks celery, chopped
1/2 cup crumbled bleu cheese
1/2 cup pecans
2 T maple syrup

In a small saucepan over medium heat, toss the pecans with the maple syrup. Cook until the syrup is absorbed and crystallizes around the pecans. Set aside to cool. Meanwhile, make the **Dijon vinaigrette** with:

1/4 cup maple syrup
1/4 cup apple cider vinegar
1/3 cup extra virgin olive oil
1 t stone ground mustard
dash salt and pepper

Whisk all ingredients together and set aside. Place the greens onto a large serving plate and top with all the salad toppings, finishing with the bleu cheese. Drizzle 1/4 cup vinaigrette over the top before serving and save the rest of the dressing for later.

## Kid Friendly Chocolate Truffles

Chocolate is notorious for containing added dairy and sugars, turning a potentially healthy treat into a dietary nightmare. But real chocolate is rich in antioxidants and contains some vital nutrients. This quick and easy recipe may not be the best sugar free snack but it is a great indulgence that provides a healthier option to the potential downfalls of a natural lifestyle.

1 cup almond, hazelnut or other natural nut butter
3/4 cup of dark chocolate bits
1 cup oats, puffed millet, or brown rice crisps (available at a health food store)
1/2 cup chopped nuts (preferably the same kind as the butter)
optional: 1/2 cup of grated chocolate

Place the nut butter and nuts in a saucepan over medium heat until softened. Add the chocolate bits and stir until softened. Quickly, stir in the grains (using one or a combo the three to make up 2/3 cup) Stir until combined. Roll into 1 inch balls and set on waxed paper until firm. Roll in the grated chocolate for a gourmet touch. Store in the fridge for up to a week. Serve cooled or at room temperature.

**Quinoa Oatmeal Cookies**

Quinoa is a versatile food, making it easy to sneak into any child's diet - or a picky adult's! This cookie recipe is a great way to make even the afternoon snack a healthy one, and most children like the polka dotted appearance the quinoa provides. Use red quinoa for a fun colorful effect, or brown quinoa for a traditional look.

1 cup butter, softened
1 cup sucanat
2 eggs
1/2 cup buttermilk
2 cups whole wheat flour
2 cups oats
2 cups quinoa, prepared according to package directions and cooled
1 cup walnuts
2 teaspoons vanilla extract
1 teaspoon baking soda
1 teaspoon baking powder
1 teaspoon cinnamon

Combine the butter and sugar until creamy. Add the eggs, one at a time, then vanilla. Next, add the dry ingredients, then the quinoa. Scoop into 1 tablespoon heaps onto a greased cookie sheet and bake at 350 degrees for 12-15 minutes. Dough can be frozen for up to 2 months. If baking from frozen, extend the cooking time by 4-5 minutes.

**Rustic Apple Blueberry Tart**

Tarts always seem so intimidating, but quick and easy rustic tarts require neither a special pan, nor the time consuming task of forming perfect edges. This delicious dessert is a snap to toss together and the kids can even do it for you while you place dinner on the table.

2 cups apple chunks
1 cup blueberries
1 prepared pie crust (can be store bought but watch for healthy fats!)
1/3 cup sucanat
3 tablespoons butter

Spread the pie crust on a parchment lined baking sheet. In a bowl, combine the butter, sucanat, apples and blueberries. Spread over the center of the crust. Begin folding the remaining outer edges over the side of the crust, covering the outer 1/3 of the fruit filling. When the crust is completely folded over, bake at 400 degrees until golden brown and the filling is hot, about 20 minutes. Serve with ice cream or fresh whipped cream.

**Easy Parfaits**

Many nutritional experts believe that breakfast (or, more appropriately, break-fast) is not the time to load the body with difficult to digest foods or strong proteins. Instead, easily digested foods and cleansing fruits help wake up the metabolism for the day's work. This recipe is perfect for those that agree, as it provides protein in an easily digestible form, with fruits and some nutritious cleansing grains. Plus, it is easy to toss together on a hectic morning!

1 cup homemade yogurt
1 cup fresh berries (blueberries, raspberries, blackberries)
1/3 cup homemade granola blend

Simply layer the ingredients, starting with yogurt and ending with berries, in 2 large parfait glasses and serve chilled.

**Lunchbox Sandwiches** are also staples in the home with little ones. They are simple to toss together, can be adjusted to any dietary preferences (i.e. vegetarian, allergen free, etc) and are easily portable. Yet, the same old peanut butter and jelly can become boring quickly, and leaves plenty of room for improvement nutritionally. Here are some classic combinations that help liven things up a bit:

- Apple Swiss (apple slices with Swiss cheese)
- Sunflower Butter and Honey (just about 1 T of honey)
- Strawberry Jam and Cream Cheese (organic of course!)
- Almond Butter and Apples (slice thin for best results)
- Turkey and Cream Cheese (for older palates, add a touch of dried herbs)
- Sunflower Butter, Raisins and Celery
- Cinnamon Cream Cheese (to 8oz cream cheese, add 1 T honey and 1 t cinnamon)
- Cashew Butter and Sliced Bananas
- California Veggie (cream cheese, sun dried tomatoes and avocado slices)
- Turkey and Green Apple with Cream Cheese
- Fruit Salad (cream cheese spread on bread with sliced apples and bananas)

# For Further Learning

Want to learn more about healthy lifestyles through Jessie's work? Try our distance learning programs, which are available for self study or through the online community accessible through membership at Vintage Remedies.

Our programs include an introductory Natural Wellness course, a Family Herbalist course and the advanced Clinical Master Herbalist program. We also offer programs specific to unique needs such as Herbalism for the Birth Professional, the Natural Skin Care Development program and the Essentials Series based Natural Living Educator.

For more details on each program, overviews are included in the next few pages and you can get complete details on our website at www.VintageRemedies.com

# Natural Wellness Course
(Our Introductory Level Program)

Are you eager to learn more about natural health? The Natural Wellness program is the perfect place to begin. This introductory enrollment program covers the essentials of herbalism, aromatherapy, nutrition, natural health philosophy, natural preparations and prevention with an emphasis on practical, effective techniques. Like all of our programs, this course teaches reliable and effective natural health from a Biblical perspective, and is completely self paced, perfect for your busy lifestyle!

The program provides 120 study hours and is typically completed in 3-5 months. Upon completion, you will have a wealth of information and ideas to transform your lifestyle into a natural, holistic one. Or, you can continue studying with us by upgrading to another course. Each of the Natural Wellness program's 8 units were taken from our other courses, which makes your transition to another course upon completion simple and effortless. Furthermore, all of the tuition you paid for the Natural Wellness program applies towards the rates for another course, so not only do the grades transfer, your money does as well!

This course is also suitable for an advanced homeschooled high schooler and fits perfectly into a single school year.

# Family Herbalist Course

Ready to completely turn your home into a healthy haven with real foods, preventative care and holistic medicine? Our completely updated and revised Family Herbalist course provides everything you need! The Family Herbalist course was our first program and remains our most popular. And now, the best is even better! We took our comprehensive program and revised the material completely, updating statistics, including new and recent advancements that have taken place since the first edition was released in 2007, and reformatting the layout to make it even more user friendly and accessible! The program now includes two textbooks: Understanding Holistic Health and Botanical Medicine in the Home as well the brand new Family Herbalist student workbook, which takes you from your first unit to completion, storing your notes, thoughts and projects.

In this program, you will learn more about herbal medicine, aromatherapy, natural health philosophy, prevention in the home and so much more! As one of our graduates, you will have all the tools you need to live a completely natural and healthy lifestyle, and pass your newly established habits along to your children. While the information is presented in a practical, easy to use format, the course is one of the most comprehensive and thorough family herbalist programs available anywhere. So, we provide the foundation you need to utilize the advanced material in a clear and straightforward manner! Our whole person, integrative approach connects modern health concerns with time tested ancient medicine and modern evidence based research, and the lengthy materia medica provided ensures competency, whether you are an attentive parent or an aspiring professional. Like all of our courses, this program teaches reliable and effective natural health from a Biblical perspective. The newly revised program contains 26 units, which are usually completed in 12-18 months. It provides 360 study hours and is self paced for your convenience.

# Herbalism for the Birth Professional

This brand new program is now available for doulas, childbirth educators, midwives and anyone else that works with childbearing women! Tailored just for your unique needs as a birth professional, this 14 unit program includes herbalism, aromatherapy, specific information for educating and empowering your clients or patients with natural solutions and even information on boosting your own immunity and protecting yourself in hospital or other high exposure situations!

Enrollment Includes:

258 page 8.5x11 spiral bound textbook
Accompanying workbook
The Handbook of Vintage Remedies (2nd edition, upon release in March)
The Vintage Remedies Guide to Real Food
Essential Oil Trio
6 months access to online learning center, grading for exams and feedback for projects

# Natural Living Educator

Are you ready to share your love of real foods and natural health with others? It's easy to become a Natural Living Educator through Vintage Remedies, and turn your passion into a profession - or expand your existing wellness career!

Our unique Essentials Series (www.VREssentials.com) can be taught only be taught by Vintage Remedies Certified Natural Living Educators. Whether you are a parent that is passionate about natural health, a care provider eager to increase the learning opportunities for your patients, a childbirth professional interested in continuing the support you offer your families or a wellness professional excited about new ways to reach your community, we've got the answer! Our certification program is thorough, yet manageable for even the busiest professional and our support staff walks with you every step of the way.

The certification process takes place entirely in the comfort of your own home - at your own pace! The program can be completed in an average of 4-6 months, but we provide a full year from your enrollment date to complete your certification! If you need an extension, those are available as well. Upon certification, our office support continues with website referrals and a special educator portal, where we provide tools and tips for success with your programs.

There are two paths to certification. The direct entry includes the Natural Wellness course materials and is perfect if you are new to Vintage Remedies. If you're already a student or graduate of our programs, you'll want to take the shorter student route, which enables you to skip the academic requirement, assuming that you've completed the required units.

# Natural Skin Care Development

Ever wondered what's in your skin care? Did you know the average individual uses over 9 different products a day with a combined total of 126 unique ingredients. Nearly 90% of those ingredients have never been evaluated for safety by any publicly accountable institution? Many of these products contain known or suspected carcinogens, pesticides, reproductive toxins and endocrine disrupters! These ingredients penetrate the skin quickly, resulting in a myriad of health concerns, including premature aging! Skip the risky products and the pricey natural spa products by making your own, customized formulations unique to your skin care needs and preferences with this 30 unit program.

This course teaches the essentials of natural skin care, herbalism and aromatherapy so that you'll have the knowledge and insight you need to correctly determine which ingredients are safe and appropriate for your needs. You'll learn all about dozens of natural ingredients, including not only how they are used in natural skin care but what to consider when selecting a supplier. And you'll put those skills to work by mastering the techniques to produce dozens of products and developing your own customized formulations.

Everything you need to become an expert at natural skin care development is right here in this brand new course! Package includes spiral bound textbook with over 300 pages of information from the chemistry of essential oils and herbalism to the best ways to create custom formulas for any situation! Also includes 1 study guide, packed with study tips, bonus material and assigned projects and tests, 1 formula workbook, which walks you through the development of your first custom formulas, and a paperback product formulas guide, which includes over 200 proven recipes for natural skin care, many of which were huge hits with Jessie's previous spa care business, and have been kept under lock and key for years! For additional technique mastery, 2 DVDs are included, which demonstrate many of the various products and formulas in a tutorial format.

# Clinical Master Herbalist

Our Clinical Master Herbalist program is designed to cover every aspect of plant medicine imaginable! In addition to learning more about herbalism, aromatherapy and nutrition, you'll learn botany and plant identification, phytochemistry, ethnobotany, and many more aspects of botanical care in this program. As a graduate, you'll enter the field of herbalism fully equipped with the training and experience necessary for success. By combining the art and science of natural medicine, as a Vintage Remedies certified Clinical Master Herbalist, you'll know how to observe, distinguish and prevent susceptibilities and patterns of disease using the holistic model of care. This whole person, integrative approach is essential to effective herbal medicine.

The course also include information on related areas of study that directly impact our health and the effectiveness and sustainability of botanical medicine, including environmental health, food history, philosophies of natural health, microbial patterns and human development. This program is ideal if you're ready to become a Clinical Master Herbalist, if you're a licensed medical professional desiring to include integrative herbalism into your existing career, or if you aspire to become a recognized professional in the field of herbalism. To fully cover the extent of this large field, it exclusively covers herbalism and those areas that are directly related to botanical medicine, and like all of our courses, comes from a Biblical perspective. An emphasis is placed on relevant, current health concerns and up to date scientific evidence, placing you, as a Clinical Master Herbalist, at the cutting edge of the field!

The program includes a total of 68 units, which provide 1400 hours of study and is typically completed in 3-4 years.

# About The Author

Jessie Hawkins founded Vintage Remedies to answer the growing need of women and parents everywhere to have a reliable source to turn to for answers to their natural health questions. What began as a small consulting practice blossomed into multiple written works, an extensive website filled with tips and formulas for natural living distance study programs and the Essentials Series, all of which educate individuals around the world on the safe and appropriate use of natural options in the home.

When she is not consulting, writing or speaking, Jessie stays busy with her husband and their four children in a Nashville suburb they call home.

**Other Works by Jessie:**

*Vintage Remedies for Tweens*
*The Vintage Remedies Guide to Real Food*
*The Vintage Remedies Guide to Bread*
*The Kitchen Herbal*
*Real Foods on a Budget*
*Vintage Remedies Study Courses and Curricula*

Find Jessie Online:

blog.JessieHawkins.com
VintageRemedies.com

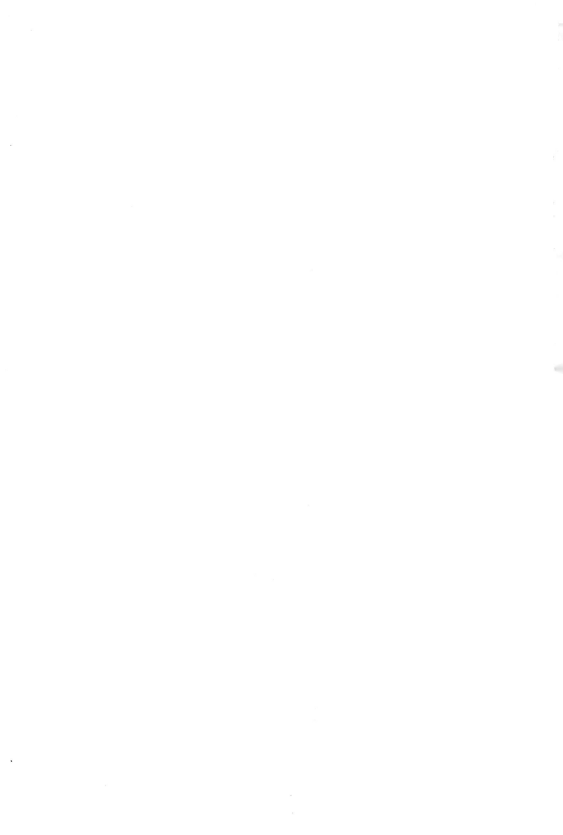